Pharmacology Made Easy, Volume 1

Callie Parker

Copyright © 2025 by Callie Parker

All rights reserved.

No portion of this book may be reproduced in any form without written permission from the publisher or author, except as permitted by U.S. copyright law.

🎉 **Wait!** Before You Dive In... Grab Your **FREE** Nursing Study Survival Kit! 🎉

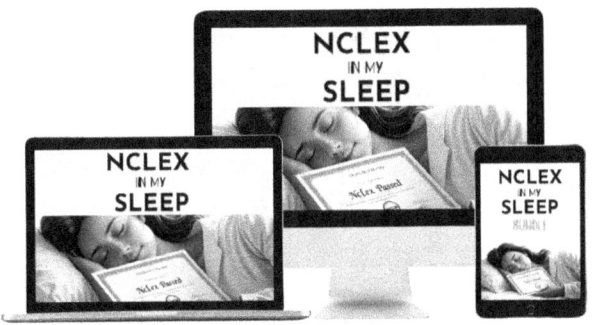

Nursing school is no joke—that's why **MadeEasy.Academy** is committed to sending the ladder back down and rescuing those of you in the trenches!

Ready to study smarter, not harder? We've got exactly what you need.

Your FREE NCLEX in My Sleep Bundle Includes:

✅ **Who's Dying First?** The Prioritization Playbook: Because patient safety is kind of a big deal. 😬

✅ **Flashcard Frenzy: Memorize or Die Trying:** Pre-made Anki cards to save your sanity.

✅ **WTF Does This Lab Value Mean?** Cheat Sheet: No more second-guessing normal vs. "oh sh*t" levels.

✅ **NCLEX Mnemonics That Stick (Like Tape on an IV Line):** Memory hacks you'll actually remember.

✅ **Med Math Without the Mental Breakdown:** Because no one wants to commit a dosage error. 💀

 Head over to **MadeEasy.Academy** to grab your bundle. Let's turn nursing school stress into success!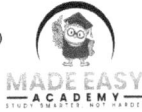

But that's not all...
🎁 BONUS 🎁

Your Bundle Includes an Exclusive 50% OFF Discount Code for your next course at Made Easy Academy
(Launching April 1!)

At **MadeEasy.Academy** we don't just simplify nursing—we transform it into an effortless, memorable study process.

For each topic, you'll follow our **step by step success guide:**

Step 1. Grab your cheat sheet: All key points, zero fluff.

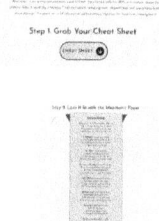

Step 2. Read your mnemonic poem: Clever rhymes to make information stick.

Step 3. Take your fill-in-the-blank quiz: Test your recall without the overwhelm.

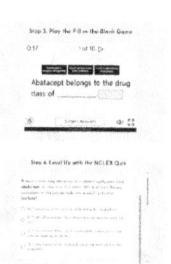

Step 4. Complete your NCLEX challenge: Realistic practice questions with clear rationales.

Step 5. Walk Into the NCLEX Like a Boss: Confident, prepared, and ready to pass.

Right now, we're laser-focused on Pharmacology, but we'll soon expand into other crucial nursing topics! Have a topic you want us to cover next? Shoot us an email at **hello@madeeasy.academy**—*we've got you!*

Contents

1. Albuterol (Proventil, Ventolin) — 7
2. Allopurinol (Zyloprim) — 9
3. Alprazolam (Xanax) — 11
4. Amitriptyline (Elavil) — 13
5. Amlodipine (Norvasc) — 15
6. Amoxicillin (Amoxil) — 17
7. Amoxicillin/Clavulanate (Augmentin) — 19
8. Amphetamine/Dextroamphetamine (Adderall) — 21
9. Apixaban (Eliquis) — 23
10. Aspirin (Bayer, Ecotrin) — 25
11. Atenolol (Tenormin) — 27
12. Atorvastatin (Lipitor) — 29
13. Azithromycin (Zithromax) — 31
14. Budesonide/Formoterol (Symbicort) — 33
15. Bupropion (Wellbutrin, Zyban) — 35
16. Buspirone (Buspar) — 37
17. Carvedilol (Coreg) — 39
18. Celecoxib (Celebrex) — 41
19. Cephalexin (Keflex) — 43
20. Cetirizine (Zyrtec) — 45

21.	Cholecalciferol (Vitamin D3)	47
22.	Citalopram (Celexa)	49
23.	Clonazepam (Klonopin)	51
24.	Clonidine (Catapres)	53
25.	Clopidogrel (Plavix)	55
26.	Cyclobenzaprine (Flexeril)	57
27.	Diclofenac (Voltaren)	59
28.	Diltiazem (Cardizem, Tiazac)	61
29.	Doxycycline (Vibramycin)	63
30.	Dulaglutide (Trulicity)	65
31.	Duloxetine (Cymbalta)	67
32.	Empagliflozin (Jardiance)	69
33.	Ergocalciferol (Vitamin D2)	71
34.	Escitalopram (Lexapro)	73
35.	Estradiol (Estrace, Climara, Vivelle-Dot)	75
36.	Ethinyl Estradiol/Norethindrone (Loestrin, etc.)	77
37.	Ethinyl Estradiol/Norgestimate (Ortho Tri-Cyclen, etc.)	79
38.	Ezetimibe (Zetia)	81
39.	Famotidine (Pepcid)	83
40.	Fenofibrate (Tricor)	85
41.	Finasteride (Proscar, Propecia)	87
42.	Fluoxetine (Prozac)	89
43.	Fluticasone (Flonase, Flovent)	91
44.	Fluticasone/Salmeterol (Advair Diskus)	93
45.	Folic Acid (Vitamin B9)	95
46.	Furosemide (Lasix)	97
47.	Gabapentin (Neurontin)	99
48.	Glimepiride (Amaryl)	101

49. Glipizide (Glucotrol) — 103
50. Hydrochlorothiazide (Microzide) — 105
51. Hydrocodone/Acetaminophen (Norco, Vicodin, Lortab) — 107
52. Hydroxyzine (Vistaril, Atarax) — 109
53. Ibuprofen (Advil, Motrin) — 111
54. Insulin Aspart (NovoLog) — 113
55. Insulin Glargine (Lantus, Basaglar) — 116
56. Insulin Lispro (Humalog, Admelog) — 118
57. Lamotrigine (Lamictal) — 120
58. Latanoprost (Xalatan) — 123
59. Levothyroxine (Synthroid, Levoxyl, Euthyrox) — 125
60. Lisdexamfetamine (Vyvanse) — 128
61. Lisinopril (Prinivil, Zestril) — 131
62. Lisinopril / Hydrochlorothiazide (Zestoretic) — 133
63. Loratadine (Claritin) — 136
64. Lorazepam (Ativan) — 138
65. Losartan (Cozaar) — 141
66. Losartan / Hydrochlorothiazide (Hyzaar) — 143
67. Meloxicam (Mobic) — 145
68. Metformin (Glucophage) — 147
69. Methylphenidate (Ritalin, Concerta) — 149
70. Metoprolol (Lopressor, Toprol XL) — 152
71. Montelukast (Singulair) — 154
72. Naproxen (Aleve, Naprosyn) — 156
73. Olmesartan (Benicar) — 158
74. Omeprazole (Prilosec) — 160
75. Ondansetron (Zofran) — 162
76. Oxycodone (Roxicodone, OxyContin, Percocet) — 164

77. Pantoprazole (Protonix) — 166
78. Paroxetine (Paxil) — 168
79. Potassium Chloride (Klor-Con, K-Dur, Micro-K) — 170
80. Pravastatin (Pravachol) — 172
81. Prednisone (Deltasone) — 174
82. Pregabalin (Lyrica) — 176
83. Propranolol (Inderal) — 178
84. Quetiapine (Seroquel) — 180
85. Rivaroxaban (Xarelto) — 183
86. Rosuvastatin (Crestor) — 185
87. Semaglutide (Ozempic, Wegovy, Rybelsus) — 187
88. Sertraline (Zoloft) — 190
89. Simvastatin (Zocor) — 192
90. Sitagliptin (Januvia) — 194
91. Spironolactone (Aldactone) — 196
92. Sumatriptan (Imitrex) — 198
93. Tamsulosin (Flomax) — 200
94. Tizanidine (Zanaflex) — 202
95. Topiramate (Topamax) — 204
96. Tramadol (Ultram) — 206
97. Trazodone (Desyrel, Oleptro) — 208
98. Triamcinolone (Kenalog, Nasacort, Aristocort) — 210
99. Venlafaxine (Effexor, Effexor XR) — 212
100. Warfarin (Coumadin) — 214

WHY Made Easy Works

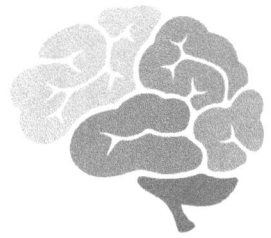

Backed by Brain Science

Let's face it — nursing school can feel like trying to drink from a firehose. Between the jargon, the never-ending lists, and the sheer volume of information, it's easy to feel overwhelmed. That's exactly why the Made Easy series was born: to make the hard stuff stick without frying your brain. And while it might look fun and playful on the outside (hello, rhymes!), it's all built on rock-solid research from the nerdy world of educational psychology.

1. COGNITIVE LOAD THEORY

First up: Cognitive Load Theory. Fancy name, simple idea — your brain can only handle so much at once. When materials are too dense or packed with fluff, your working memory taps out. Educational psychologist John Sweller figured this out, and we took notes. That's why our poems give you the essentials only, in small, memorable doses. Less clutter, more clarity. (Sweller, 1988; Clark et al., 2006)

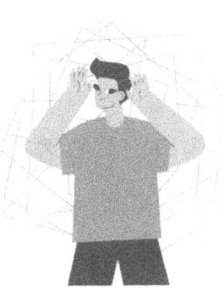

2. DUAL CODING THEORY

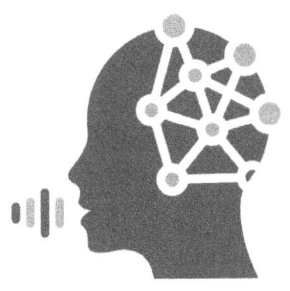

Then there's Dual Coding Theory, brought to us by Allan Paivio. He discovered that we remember things better when we learn them through both words and visuals. Our poems lean into this by using rhyme and rhythm to boost verbal memory — and bolded key terms, color coding, and clean formatting to give your visual brain a treat. Two paths to your brain = double the retention. (Paivio, 1986; Mayer, 2009)

3. ADVANCE ORGANIZERS

Psychologist David Ausubel believed that when we know how new info fits into what we already know, we learn faster. That's the beauty of our repeatable poem structure. Once you get the hang of the format, your brain relaxes — and focuses on what actually matters: the content. Think of it like a familiar playlist for your mind. (Ausubel, 1960)

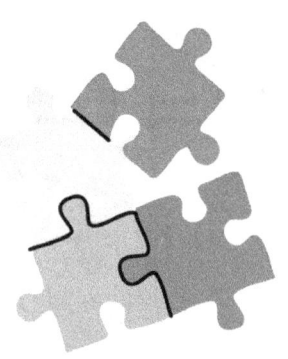

4. MICROLEARNING

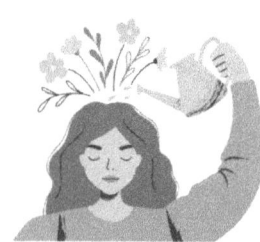

Our poems are also bite-sized by design, and that's no accident. Welcome to the world of microlearning — the idea that small, focused learning units are easier to digest and retain. This is a game-changer for busy, burnt-out students. Instead of cramming for hours, you can study just one medication, one skill, or one critical concept at a time. Snack-sized studying with full-course impact. (Hug, 2005; van den Berg & van den Berg, 2021)

5. SPACED REPETITION & RETRIEVAL PRACTICE

Last but definitely not least: spaced repetition and retrieval practice. These two learning powerhouses have proven time and again that the more often you recall information over time, the longer you'll remember it. Our poems are made for this. Easy to reread, perfect for flashcards, and fun enough to come back to (yes, we admitted it). Rinse and repeat — and retain. (Dunlosky et al., 2013)

So, yes — this method might look different than your typical textbook grind. That's the point. It's effective on purpose. Because learning tough topics shouldn't feel impossible. It should feel doable. Even a little fun. And with Made Easy, it totally is.

Read it. Rhyme it. Remember it.

That's the Made Easy Method—a simple but powerful approach to mastering complex nursing material.

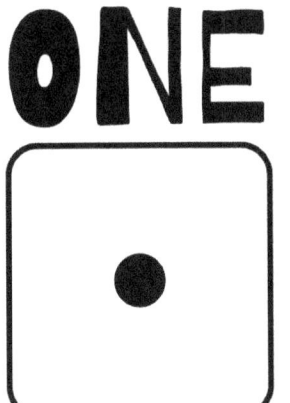

ONE

THIS ISN'T REGULAR POETRY— IT'S PURPOSEFUL

These poems weren't made to be skimmed or read once.
They're built for memory. They're built for you.

They might feel dense at first. You might pause. That's okay.
You're supposed to wrestle with the words.
It's in that wrestling—the rereading, the out-loud reciting, the highlighting—that retention starts to kick in.

Let the rhythm do the heavy lifting.
Rhyme and repetition are memory's **best** friends.
This poetry is built for practice, not perfection.

COLOR-CODE FOR CLARITY

To help you organize and absorb the content, we recommend using a color-coded system while you read.

Highlight or mark up key details with consistent colors for:

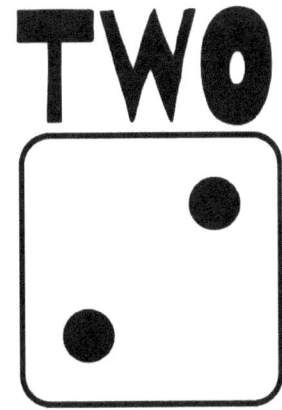

TWO

- 🟦 Drug Classification & Names
- 🟦 Mechanism of Action
- 🟦 Indications
- 🟦 Side Effects & Adverse Reactions
- 🟦 Nursing Considerations
- ▢ Monitoring Requirements
- 🟦 Patient & Caregiver Teaching Points
- ⬤ Black Box Warnings
- Pediatric Considerations
- ⬤ Drug Interactions

When you revisit the poem, your highlights will guide your recall and make review sessions faster and easier.

THREE

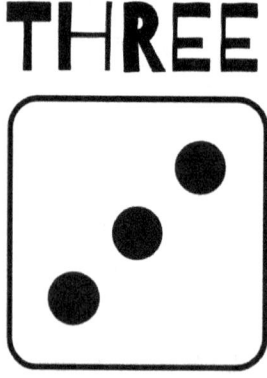

TEST WHAT YOU KNOW

After each section, you'll find a QR code that takes you straight to a short NCLEX-style quiz hosted in Google Forms. These aren't just random practice questions — they're carefully crafted to test the most important takeaways from what you just read. But the real magic? <u>The rationales.</u> Whether you get the answer right or wrong, the quiz walks you through the why. Understanding the reasoning behind each answer helps you think like a nurse, not just a test-taker.

It's not about memorizing — it's about making connections, strengthening critical thinking, and applying your knowledge in real clinical scenarios. So take your time, review the rationales, and let them guide you from confusion to clarity.

So don't just read these pages—
interact with them.

☐ **Re**ad it.

🎵 **Rhy**me it.

🧠 **Re**mem**ber** it.

That's how we make nursing Made Easy.

> "Nursing is an art: and if it is to be made an art, it requires an exclusive devotion as hard a preparation as any painter's or sculptor's work.
> - Florence Nightingale

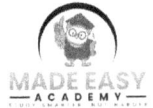

Albuterol (Proventil, Ventolin)

Beta-2 Agonist (Bronchodilator)

A bronchodilator, short-acting too,
Beta-2 agonist—it's quick to break through.
Relaxes **smooth muscles**, the **airway expands**,
Opens the **bronchi** with magical hands.

It's used for **asthma, wheezing, tight chest**,
And **COPD** when you can't catch your breath.
It's **rescue**, not daily—short bursts when you need,
A **puff** or a **neb** to help you breathe freed.

But **tachycardia** may follow its trail,
And **tremors** or **nervousness**—these might prevail.
Palpitations, headache, or **jittery** feels,
Even **hypokalemia** can be real.

Before you give, **check heart rate** and **lungs**,
Is there **improvement** when breathing is sung?
Inhale deeply, hold it in tight,
Teach them to **rinse** after each fight.

Black box? No, it doesn't hold that claim,

But still needs **caution** with **heart that's inflamed**.

Too much can lead to **paradoxical strain**,

So **monitor use** and **control** the game.

It clashes with **MAOIs** and some **beta blockers**,

May mute the magic or cause wild shockers.

Keep an eye on **potassium**, watch for the signs,

Especially in those on **diuretics** lines.

So nurses take note—this med's fast and bold,

Relief in a puff, when the breath turns cold.

Educate wisely, assess with care,

Albuterol helps when there's **no air to spare**.

Allopurinol (Zyloprim)

Antigout medication

A **xanthine oxidase inhibitor**, neat,
It **lowers uric acid**, not quick but sweet.
Prevents the build-up, not for acute gout,
But for **chronic control**, it helps smooth things out.

Used in **gout**, **kidney stones**, **tumor lysis** too,
Where **uric acid levels** wildly accrue.
It stops the **enzyme xanthine** in its track,
So purines break down with **less uric attack**.

But watch for **rash**, sometimes **severe**,
Stevens-Johnson syndrome—that's a real fear.
Also **GI upset, diarrhea, nausea**,
And rare but deadly **bone marrow aplasia**.

Before you give it, check **renal labs**,
Liver enzymes, too—look for drabs.
Uric acid levels are key to track,
And **CBC** to watch bone marrow's back.

Black Box Warning? Not on the sheet,

But reactions can still knock you off your feet.

Hypersensitivity syndrome is real—

Fever, **rash**, and **organ** ordeal.

Avoid with **azathioprine, mercaptopurine**,

It blocks their clearance and could cause ruin.

Ampicillin may cause **rashes to spike**,

So watch what they take and what they like.

Teach patients to **stay hydrated, take with food**,

To lower **GI upset** and help the mood.

Let them know this drug's not quick—

It takes **weeks** for relief to **truly stick**.

Report any **rash**, or **fever** at all,

It may be mild—or a dangerous call.

So nurses beware, and patients too,

With **allopurinol**, caution gets you through.

Alprazolam (Xanax)

Benzodiazepine

A **benzodiazepine**, calming and quick,
It works in the **CNS**—a **GABA**-based trick.
Enhances inhibition, slows down the storm,
Bringing the anxious back into form.

Used for **anxiety**, **panic attacks**,
When life's too heavy and courage lacks.
Short-term relief when emotions fly,
But not for forever—addiction runs high.

Watch for **drowsiness**, **dizziness**, too,
Confusion, fatigue, and **memory skew**.
Depression, slurred speech, or **low BP**,
Even **respiratory depression**, you see.

Before you give, **assess their mood**,
And **CNS status**—don't misconstrue.
Check **vital signs**, especially **rate**,
Respiratory checks help mitigate fate.

Black Box Warning: a serious one,
Combined with **opioids**, damage is done.
Risk of **sedation**, **coma**, and death—
Monitor breathing and depth of breath.

Don't mix with alcohol, it adds to the toll,
And **CYP3A4 inhibitors** may play a role.
Drugs like **ketoconazole**, **clarithromycin** too,
Can raise its levels and worsen the view.

Teach the patient: **don't stop abruptly**,
Taper off slowly and do it subtly.
Warn about driving or heavy machine,
Until they know how it makes them feel keen.

Lock it away—**controlled substance class four**,
Risk of **dependence** behind that door.
Short-term use with nursing eyes near,
Alprazolam brings calm—and sometimes fear.

Amitriptyline (Elavil)

Tricyclic antidepressant

A **tricyclic antidepressant**, old but strong,
It's been on the shelves for **decades long**.
Blocks reuptake of **norepinephrine** and **serotonin** too,
To **lift low moods** and **change the view**.

Used for **depression**, **neuropathic pain**,
Fibromyalgia, or **migraines** that strain.
Sometimes for **insomnia** or **anxiety's grip**,
But start off **low**—it's a potent script.

Watch for **sedation**, it kicks in fast,
Dry mouth, **blurred vision**, these symptoms last.
Constipation, **urinary retention** arise,
And **orthostatic hypotension** may catch by surprise.

There's risk for **weight gain**, and **sweating** too,
And **cardiac issues** that might ensue.
QT prolongation, arrhythmia flare—
Monitor **EKGs** with cardiac care.

Before you give it, **check mental state**,
Watch for **suicide risk** that could escalate.
Elderly? Be cautious—they're more at risk,
For **falls, confusion**, and side effects brisk.

Yes, there's a **Black Box Warning** you should know:
Suicidal thoughts can start to grow.
Especially in **teens and young adults**,
So monitor moods, results, and faults.

It interacts with **MAOIs**—a big red flag,
Can trigger **serotonin syndrome** or drag.
Also avoid with **anticholinergics** in tow,
Or **CNS depressants** that further slow.

Teach patients it takes **weeks to kick in**,
And stopping too fast? A withdrawal spin.
Avoid **alcohol, rise slowly**, and stay alert,
This med helps heal—but misuse can hurt.

Amlodipine (Norvasc)

Calcium Channel Blocker (Antihypertensive)

A **calcium channel blocker**, smooth and slow,
It helps the **blood pressure** gently flow.
Blocks **calcium influx** in vessels' walls,
So the **arteries relax**, and **pressure falls**.

Used for **hypertension, angina pain**,
And **CAD**—when there's vascular strain.
It helps the heart do **less workload**, more rest,
A daily med to keep hearts at their best.

Watch for **peripheral edema** first,
Dizziness, fatigue, and **flushing burst**.
Palpitations may show up too,
And **hypotension** is something to view.

Before you give, **check BP and heart rate**,
Hold the dose if **systolic's too late**.
If **heart rate is low**, like **under 60**,
Call the provider—it's better to be picky.

No Black Box Warning, but don't take it light—
If used with **beta-blockers**, keep insight.
May **worsen angina** if stopped too fast,
So **taper slowly**—let withdrawal pass.

Avoid with **grapefruit**, it raises the risk,
And **CYP3A4 inhibitors** can also twist.
Use caution with **liver disease**,
Lower doses may better please.

Teach them to report **swelling in legs**,
And **chest pain** that flares or **dizziness** begs.
Rise **slowly**, watch for the **drop**,
Stay on track and **don't just stop**.

So with **Norvasc**, keep the vessel tone,
And teach your patients what's unknown.
A calm, cool ride for the pressure fight,
Amlodipine keeps the numbers right.

Amoxicillin (Amoxil)

Penicillin antibiotic

A **penicillin antibiotic**, classic and true,
Broad-spectrum power in a capsule for you.
It stops **cell wall synthesis**, bacteria burst,
By blocking **peptidoglycan**—a microbial curse.

Used for **infections**—**ear**, **nose**, and **throat**,
UTIs, **skin**, and **bronchitis** it wrote.
Also for **sinus** and **dental pain**,
And **H. pylori** in ulcers' domain.

But **nausea**, **vomiting**, **diarrhea** may show,
And **rash** or **itching** from head to toe.
C. diff infection is a risk that's real,
So assess for **bloody stools** and how they feel.

Watch for **allergic reactions** fast—
Anaphylaxis can hit like a blast.
Hives, **swelling**, or trouble breathing in,
Call a code—don't wait to begin.

No **Black Box Warning**, but still beware,

Of **superinfections**—so nurses care.

Yeast may bloom where flora fade,

So teach them signs where balance strayed.

Check for **allergies** to **penicillin** base,

Or **cephalosporins**—they're in the same race.

Use caution with **warfarin**—bleeding may rise,

And **methotrexate** levels may surprise.

Teach them to **finish the full course**, not just some,

Even if **symptoms are starting to numb**.

Take with or without **food**, it's okay,

But report **rash** or **itch** without delay.

So **Amoxicillin**, with power and might,

Fights the bugs and helps things right.

A nurse's ally—when used with grace,

Track reactions, labs, and healing pace.

Amoxicillin/Clavulanate (Augmentin)

Combination antibiotic

A duo med with double the might
Beta-lactam power for the infection fight.
Amoxicillin blocks the **bacterial wall**,
While **clavulanate** makes resistance fall.
It's a **penicillin combo**, broad and bold,
Treats infections that are hard to hold.
Respiratory, UTIs, skin, and **ears**,
Even **sinus, bites**, and **lung-based fears**.

Clavulanate stops **beta-lactamase** foes,
So **amoxicillin** can land its blows.
Together they tackle **resistant strains**,
When plain penicillin goes down the drains.
Expect **diarrhea, nausea, GI upset**,
And **rash** that could be a bigger threat.
Yeast infections, headache, liver strain,
And rare **C. diff** might cause bowel pain.

No **Black Box Warning**, but still use care—
Watch for **anaphylaxis** out of nowhere.
Hives, swelling, wheezing may arise,
Always check for **allergy ties**.
Before you give it, **check liver labs**,
And watch for signs if their **joints feel drab**.
ALT, AST might elevate,
So **monitor function** before it's too late.

Caution with **warfarin**, bleeding may spike,
And **methotrexate** may not act right.
Don't give with **allopurinol**, rash could ignite,
Watch for **probenecid**—it alters the fight.
Teach patients to **take with food** to ease the gut,
And **complete the course**, no matter what.
Warn of **diarrhea** and **signs of yeast**,
And to call if **rash** or **itching** has increased.

So **Augmentin** joins the med parade,
When **simple penicillin** starts to fade.
With **clavulanate**, it breaks through shields—
A nurse's tool for resistant fields.

Amphetamine/Dextroamphetamine (Adderall)

Central nervous system stimulant

A **CNS stimulant**, strong and fast,
It helps **focus** and **attention** last.
Two parts working in synergy tight—
Amphetamine and **dextro**, both ignite.
It **boosts dopamine and norepinephrine**,
In the **prefrontal cortex**, where thoughts begin.
Used for **ADHD** and **narcolepsy's sway**,
To sharpen the brain and stay awake all day.

But side effects can pack a punch:
Insomnia, **irritability**, skipping lunch.
Tachycardia, **palpitations** may rise,
And **elevated BP** is no surprise.
May cause **weight loss**, **dry mouth**, **mood swing**,
And **tics**, **anxiety**, or a jittery zing.
In rare cases, **psychosis** may appear—
Hallucinations, paranoia, fear.

Before you give, **check heart rate and BP**,
And screen for **mental health history**.
Avoid in those with **cardiac disease**,
And watch for **substance misuse** with ease.
There's a **Black Box Warning**—don't ignore:
Abuse potential—controlled **Schedule II** for sure.
Dependence, **addiction**, even **death**,
Especially if mixed or taken in excess breath.

It interacts with **MAOIs**—dangerous pair,
Can lead to **hypertensive crisis**—so beware.
Use caution with **antacids**, they change absorption,
And with other **stimulants**, there's overstimulation.
Teach patients to **take it early**, not late,
To avoid **insomnia** and a restless state.
Encourage **nutrition**, **hydration** too,
And **monitor weight**—that's smart to do.

So nurses note this stimulant's might,
Great when used with judgment right.
For focus, drive, and mental pace,
Adderall can hold its place.

Apixaban (Eliquis)

Direct oral anticoagulant

A **Factor Xa inhibitor**, sleek and direct,
It stops **clot formation**, keeps vessels in check.
An **anticoagulant**, modern and clean,
No need for **INR** like warfarin's routine.
Used to prevent **DVT** and **PE**,
For **non-valvular A-fib**, it sets clots free.
After **hip or knee surgery**, it's also shown,
To keep the risk of thrombosis low.

But with this med, **bleeding leads**—
From **bruising** to GI or **nosebleed feeds**.
Hematomas, hematuria, and **stool that's black**,
All signs the dose may need to back.
There's a **Black Box Warning**—take great care,
Spinal hematomas may occur out there.
If they've had a **neuraxial block**,
That bleeding risk deserves a talk.

Also risk if **stopped too soon**,
A **clot rebound** may come too soon.

Always confirm they're **bridging right**,

So no surprise stroke comes to light.

Check **renal function**, adjust with age,

In **hepatic impairment**, assess the stage.

No **antidote** for a while was known,

But now there's **andexanet alfa** shown.

Avoid with drugs that **raise bleed risk**,

Like **NSAIDs**, **SSRIs**, or **antiplatelet disks**.

And if on **strong CYP3A4 inhibitors**,

The bleed risk climbs—warn the visitors.

Teach patients to **take twice daily**, as planned,

Don't **double doses**, or bleeding's at hand.

Let dentists know before they clean,

And **fall risks** must be clearly seen.

So **Eliquis** flows through modern care,

A clot-prevention tool with flair.

But nurses must watch each **bleeding clue**,

Because small signs can lead to something new.

Aspirin (Bayer, Ecotrin)

NSAID/antiplatelet

A classic **NSAID**, still standing tall,
Antiplatelet, **analgesic**, it does it all.
It blocks **COX-1** and **COX-2** in the track,
Stopping **prostaglandins** and **platelet clump** back.
Used for **pain**, **fever**, and **inflammation**,
And low-dose for **clot prevention** in circulation.
Helps prevent **stroke**, **MI**, and **TIAs**,
A heart hero in many ways.

Side effects? Well, there's a list:
GI upset tops the twist.
Ulcers, **heartburn**, and **nausea** too,
And **bleeding** risk that's real and true.
There's **tinnitus** with high doses—ringing that sings,
And **Reye's syndrome** in kids—serious things.
Bruising, **petechiae**, and blood that won't clot,
Are nursing signs you must have caught.

Before you give, **assess for bleeds**,
Past **ulcers**, **surgery**, or **liver needs**.

Check **platelets**, **H&H**, and more,

Especially if they're bleeding from the floor.

There **is a Black Box Warning**, be advised:

For **GI bleeding** and **ulcer risk**—sized.

Also **risk of stroke or MI** if misused,

Especially when not properly fused.

Avoid with **anticoagulants**—that's key,

And **NSAIDs, alcohol**, or **Ginkgo tea**.

Interactions can **raise the bleed**,

So watch the full **med list** and proceed.

Teach to **take with food**, not on an empty plate,

And not to **crush enteric-coated**, it seals their fate.

Hold before **surgery**, typically **a week**,

To let platelets recover their normal peak.

In kids, say no unless the doc insists—

Reye's syndrome risk still exists.

So **Aspirin**, though humble, must be known,

For **nurses**, it's a cornerstone.

Atenolol (Tenormin)

Beta-blocker (antihypertensive)

A **beta-blocker**, cardio-selective in tone,
It slows the heart and calms it down alone.
Blocks beta-1 receptors with care,
So the **heart rate drops**, less pressure to bear.
Used for **hypertension**, **angina pain**,
Post-MI, it helps the heart maintain.
Also used for **arrhythmias** in stride,
To keep that beat from slipping wide.

But side effects you need to chart:
Bradycardia, too slow a heart.
Fatigue, **cold extremities**, and **dizzy heads**,
Sometimes **depression**, and heavy like lead.
In **diabetics**, use caution, friend—
It may **mask hypoglycemia's** trend.
No shaky hands, no racing heart,
Just low sugar signs that don't depart.

Check heart rate and BP before each dose,
If **heart rate is under 60**, then don't get close.

Also check for **CHF signs**, it may mask the rise—
Weight gain, crackles, or swollen thighs.
There's a **Black Box Warning**, nurses beware:
Abrupt withdrawal? Don't you dare.
Can lead to **chest pain**, even **MI**,
So **taper it slowly**, don't make them cry.

Avoid with **calcium channel blockers** too,
Like **verapamil**, the pressure might stew.
Watch for **digoxin**, the rhythm can slow,
So keep an eye on that cardiac flow.
Teach patients to **take it each day**,
Same time, with or without food on the tray.
Tell them to **rise slow**, orthostatic is real,
And report **fatigue** they constantly feel.

So **Atenolol**—steady, slow, and wise,
Tames the heart so no surprise.
But with power comes nursing grace,
To keep the rhythm in its place.

Atorvastatin (Lipitor)
Statin

A **statin** drug that's strong and slick,
It lowers **lipids** nice and quick.
It **inhibits HMG-CoA reductase**, the key,
The **liver makes less cholesterol**—you see?

Used for **hyperlipidemia**, high **LDL**,
Prevention of stroke, **MI** as well.
For **cardiac risk**, it's a go-to med,
Keeps **plaques** from growing, keeps **clots** in check instead.

But watch for **headache, GI pain**,
And **muscle aches** that might remain.
Myopathy is the term to know,
And worse—**rhabdomyolysis** can grow.

Check for **liver damage**—that's the cue,
AST and **ALT**—review those, too.
Liver failure, though rare, can arise,
So **monitor labs** and look for signs.

No Black Box Warning, but be on guard,

With **grapefruit juice**, it hits too hard.

CYP3A4 inhibitors make it rise,

So avoid strong meds that **interact** in disguise.

Pregnancy? Stop! It's a firm "no,"

It's **Category X**—risk too high to show.

Also avoid in **liver disease**,

And in **breastfeeding**—just say, "please."

Teach to take it at **night**, that's best,

When **cholesterol synthesis** gets no rest.

Report **muscle pain**, **weakness**, or **fatigue**,

And **limit alcohol**, don't overindulge league.

So **Lipitor** helps the vessels stay wide,

But nurses must **monitor** and guide.

With labs, checks, and teaching clear,

We keep the heart safe—year to year.

Azithromycin (Zithromax)
Macrolide antibiotic

A **macrolide antibiotic**, smooth and long,
It fights **bacterial infections** strong.
It **inhibits protein synthesis**, ribosome bind,
Stops bacteria from growing, leaving none behind.

Used for **respiratory**, **ear**, and **skin**,
STIs, **strep throat**, and **sinus within**.
Chlamydia, **pneumonia**, **bronchitis**, too—
One pill a day, and you're pushing through.

But side effects can still arise:
GI upset, not a surprise.
Nausea, **diarrhea**, **cramping** pains,
And **QT prolongation** in heart's refrains.

Though rare, there's risk of **liver strain**,
Watch for **jaundice** or **abdominal pain**.
Hearing loss at high doses might be seen,
And **C. diff colitis** may intervene.

Check their **EKG** if they're at risk,
With **cardiac meds**, you must not miss.
Monitor **LFTs** if they're on long-term,
And **renal function** if concerns confirm.

No **Black Box Warning**, but don't go blind—
There are **serious interactions** to keep in mind.
Avoid with other **QT-prolonging** drugs,
Or **antacids** that bind and give it shrugs.

Teach them to **take it with food** if GI's tight,
And to **avoid aluminum/magnesium at night**.
Tell them it's okay to take once a day,
But **finish the course**, don't go halfway.

So **Zithromax** is handy, with dosing so light,
But nurses must guide to use it right.
With heart, gut, and labs in view,
Azithromycin gets the job through.

Budesonide/Formoterol (Symbicort)

Combination corticosteroid and long-acting beta agonist

A combo med with dual control,

To help the lungs breathe strong and whole.

Budesonide's a **steroid**, calm and slow,

While **Formoterol**, a **LABA**, helps airflow.

It's an **inhaled corticosteroid + long-acting beta-2**,

Reduces **inflammation** and opens you through.

Used for **asthma** and **COPD**,

Not for **rescue**, but for **therapy**.

Budesonide tames the **swelling and flame**,

While Formoterol opens the **bronchial frame**.

Together they **prevent exacerbation**,

And improve daily **respiration**.

Side effects? Well, take a peek:

Thrush, **hoarseness**, or a **voice that's weak**.

Headache, **tremor**, or **palpitations**,

And **infections** in **respiratory stations**.

No **Black Box Warning** for both combined,
But **LABAs alone**? Risk is outlined.
They may **raise death risk** if taken solo,
So always combine—don't let that flow go.
Before you give, **check lungs and rate**,
Listen for **wheezes** and breathing state.
Teach to **rinse the mouth** after each puff,
To prevent **candidiasis**—that stuff's rough.

Avoid with other **beta-agonist** meds,
And use caution if **heart disease** treads.
It may interact with **diuretics**, too,
And cause **hypokalemia** to sneak through.
Teach patients to take it **every day**,
Even when **symptoms fade away**.
Not for **rescue**, that's key to know—
They'll need **albuterol** if airflow won't flow.

So **Symbicort** helps the lungs stay wide,
With **prevention and balance** side by side.
A daily dose with nurse insight,
Keeps **asthma** and **COPD** more light.

Bupropion (Wellbutrin, Zyban)
Atypical antidepressant

An **atypical antidepressant**, quite unique,
It lifts the mood and boosts your peak.
It **blocks reuptake** of **dopamine** and **norepinephrine**,
A different path than **SSRIs** have been.
Used for **depression** and **SAD** (seasonal kind),
And to help with **smoking cessation**—reclaim your mind.
Marketed as **Wellbutrin** to lift the gray,
Or **Zyban** to make the smokes go away.

But with this med, side effects can show:
Dry mouth, **nausea**, and **anxiety's** flow.
Insomnia is common—take it **early in day**,
To help the brain, not make sleep stray
The biggest risk? A **seizure event**,
Especially if dosing is not well spent.
There's a **Black Box Warning**, don't forget:
Suicidal thoughts in youth are a threat.

Avoid in those with **seizure disorder**,
Or **eating disorders**—that's a firm order.

Also not for those withdrawing **alcohol**,

Or **benzos**—seizure risk could appall.

Before you give, assess **mental state**,

And for **bipolar disorder**, investigate.

It can cause **mania** to suddenly flare,

So rule that out with nursing care.

It interacts with **MAOIs**, that's bad—

A **two-week gap** is to be had.

Also caution with **levodopa, ritonavir**,

And **CYP2B6** inhibitors near.

Teach patients to **swallow whole**, not crush,

And **avoid late doses**—that's a rush.

Let them know that **mood lift takes time**,

It's **weeks**, not days, before they climb.

So **Bupropion** stands apart from the rest,

In **dopamine drive**, it's one of the best.

For mood or smoke, it plays its role—

With nurse support, it helps heal whole.

Buspirone (Buspar)
Non-benzodiazepine anxiolytic

An **anxiolytic**, gentle and slow,
With **no sedation** or **addiction** to show.
It's not a **benzo**, not meant for quick,
But for **chronic anxiety**, it does the trick.

It works on **serotonin**, partial **5-HT1A**,
Altering mood in a non-sedating way.
Also nudges some **dopamine** sites,
To calm the mind without sleep's heights.

Used for **GAD**—that's **generalized fear**,
But takes **1 to 4 weeks** to fully appear.
It won't help panic or act real fast,
But for daily calm, the relief can last.

Side effects? Let's break it down:
Dizziness, **headache**, and a **spinning** crown.
Nausea, **nervousness**, and **lightheaded drift**,
But no high, no buzz, and no withdrawal shift.

No **Black Box Warning**—a lighter track,

But still, keep caution in your pack.

Use care in those with **liver strain**,

And **renal impairment** brings dosage pain.

It doesn't play nice with **MAOIs**,

That combo can make **blood pressure** rise.

Also avoid with **grapefruit juice**,

It raises levels and cuts it loose.

Teach to take it **consistently**, every day,

Not **as needed**—it doesn't work that way.

Tell them not to expect it to act like a benzo,

And no alcohol—keep that tempo.

So **Buspirone** walks a **gentle line**,

No habit formed, just peace in time.

With steady use and nurse's guide,

Anxiety can step aside.

Carvedilol (Coreg)

Alpha/beta-blocker

A **beta-blocker**, but it's more than that,
It's **nonselective**, with **alpha-block** combat.
It slows the **heart rate**, drops **BP** smooth,
And helps the heart get back in groove.
Used for **heart failure**, **hypertension**, too,
And **post-MI** to help get through.
It lowers **afterload**, protects the heart,
And gives those weak beats a better start.

Side effects you'll want to chart:
Bradycardia, **hypotension**, and a **heavy heart**.
Dizziness, **fatigue**, and feeling faint,
Orthostatic drops can make them faint.
It may mask signs of **low blood sugar**,
So in **diabetics**, be even surer.
Cold hands, **weight gain**, **SOB**—
Are signs of **worsening HF**, you see.

There's **no Black Box**, but don't miss the beat,
It must be **tapered slowly**, not on repeat.

Stopping quick can cause **chest pain**,
And lead to **MI** or **cardiac strain**.
Before you give it, **check heart rate**,
If it's under **60**, you might want to wait.
And always assess for **crackles or swelling**,
Signs that the **heart's in trouble**, compelling.

Be cautious with **digoxin**, **CCBs** like **verapamil**,
Together they might **slow the rhythm** still.
CYP2D6 inhibitors can increase effect,
So **monitor BP** and all you'd expect.
Teach patients to **rise slowly**, take with **food**,
To help with **dizziness** and **mood**.
Tell them not to skip or double dose,
And check **pulse** and **BP** at most.

So **Carvedilol**, with careful might,
Protects the heart both day and night.
But nurses must guide, assess, and teach—
To keep its benefits within safe reach.

Celecoxib (Celebrex)

COX-2 selective NSAID

A **COX-2 inhibitor**, sleek and refined,
Less **GI upset**, by design.
An **NSAID**, yes—but selective and neat,
It helps with **pain, swelling,** and **inflammatory heat.**

Used for **arthritis**, both **osteo** and **RA**,
Also **ankylosing spondylitis** may sway.
Dysmenorrhea pain? It plays a role,
With fewer **stomach ulcers** as a goal.

But don't let that safety lull you in—
There's still **risk of clotting** deep within.
MI, stroke, and **thrombotic events,**
Are serious **Black Box** contents.

Other effects may show up too:
Hypertension, edema, and **GI flu.**
Though **ulcer risk** is lower than most,
It's not completely without a host.

Use caution in those with **heart disease**,

And with **renal or liver** issues, dose with ease.

Avoid if there's a **sulfa allergy**,

Or **after CABG**—that's policy.

Check **BP** and **renal labs** before,

BUN, creatinine, and more in store.

Teach to take it **with food**, not alone,

And report if **chest pain** or **weakness** is shown.

Avoid with other **NSAIDs** or **blood thinners**,

That combo makes **bleeding** no winners.

ACE inhibitors may lose their might,

And **lithium** levels could rise overnight.

So **Celecoxib**, precise and clean,

But still, a **risky med** behind the screen.

With **nurse guidance**, safe it can be—

A balanced act of **efficacy**.

Cephalexin (Keflex)

First-Generation Cephalosporin – Antibiotic

A **cephalosporin**, first in line,
Cephalexin works just fine.
It busts up bugs that cause a mess—
Gram-positive mostly, with some **Gram-neg** success.
Used for **skin, throat,** and **UTIs,**
And **respiratory** infections on the rise.
Also treats **dental abscess pain,**
And **cellulitis** in tissue strain.

It **disrupts the bacterial cell wall,**
So the pathogen breaks down and falls.
A **bactericidal** mode of fight,
Kills the germs, not just slows them right.
Take it **with or without food,**
But **GI upset** may intrude.
So if their stomach starts to turn,
A little snack can help them learn.

Side effects? A few to know:
Nausea, vomiting, or **diarrhea flow.**

Rash or **itching**—watch that skin,
Could mean an **allergy** is creeping in.
If they've had a **penicillin scare**,
There's **cross-reactivity** to beware.
Not always, but still be wise—
Check allergy history before it flies.

Rarely, **C. diff colitis** may appear,
With **watery stool**, pain in the rear.
So teach them not to treat on hand,
But call the doc—that's the plan.
Take the **full course**, don't stop fast,
Even if they feel good at last.
Stopping early helps bugs survive,
And next time, they might just thrive.

Watch **renal function**—dose with care,
If kidneys aren't quite fully there.
Monitor **WBCs** and symptoms too,
To ensure the infection is through.

Cetirizine (Zyrtec)

Second-generation antihistamine

An **antihistamine**, second-gen,
For **allergy symptoms** again and again.
Blocks **H1 receptors**, smooth and tight,
So **histamine** can't start its fight.

Used for **rhinitis**, both **seasonal** and **chronic**,
And **urticaria**—itchy, not iconic.
Relieves the **sneezing**, **runny nose**, and **itch**,
Without the **sedation** that first-gens pitch.

Still, **drowsiness** can show in some,
Though it's less than when **diphenhydramine** comes.
Also **dry mouth**, **fatigue**, maybe **throat dry**,
And **headache** can linger and flutter by.

There's **no Black Box Warning** on this one's track,
But **renal dosing** may need to scale back.
In **older adults**, go low and slow,
To prevent **confusion** or **fall risk** below.

Before you give, **assess their signs**,

Allergy symptoms or **hives** that align.

Check for **renal function** if used long,

And ask if they're mixing it in their **daily throng**.

Interactions? Very few,

But caution with **alcohol** or a **CNS stew**.

It may cause a **synergistic sedative drift**,

Especially when given a **benzo lift**.

Teach patients it's **once a day**,

With or without food, either way.

If **drowsiness** shows, try it **at night**,

And let them know that's perfectly right.

So **Cetirizine** clears the airways clean,

A modern fix for **histamine**.

A daily helper with minimal fuss,

A nurse-approved choice for the allergy bus.

Cholecalciferol (Vitamin D3)

Vitamin

Known as **Vitamin D₃**, sunshine's delight,
It helps keep your **calcium** and **phosphate** right.
A **fat-soluble vitamin**, stored with grace,
It builds up in bones, keeping structure in place.

It's used to treat or **prevent deficiency**,
In **osteoporosis**, it works efficiently.
Also for **rickets**, **osteomalacia's** cure,
And to help **calcium absorption** endure.

Side effects are rare when dosed with care,
But too much? Then **hypercalcemia's** there.
Nausea, **vomiting**, **weakness**, and **thirst**,
Kidney stones may come—the worst.

Before you give, **check vitamin D level**,
And **serum calcium**, keep it on a level.
In **renal disease**, use wisely, dear,
As **electrolyte shifts** can soon appear.

There's **no Black Box Warning** to bring,
But it's still a supplement with a swing.
Toxicity risk when doses are high—
Especially when symptoms amplify.

Watch drug interactions if you please:
With **thiazide diuretics**, calcium may seize.
And **anticonvulsants** like **phenytoin**, too,
May lower D levels and follow through.

Teach patients to take it with **meals or fat**,
To **boost absorption**—they'll love that.
Avoid **over-the-counter D** they don't need,
And watch out for **hidden** doses in feed.

So **Cholecalciferol**, simple and bright,
Brings **bone strength** and **calcium** to light.
But nurses must monitor, dose just right—
Too much of the sun can still burn the night.

Citalopram (Celexa)

SSRI antidepressant

An **SSRI**, gentle and clean,
It boosts **serotonin** in the mental machine.
Blocks the **reuptake**, lets good vibes stay,
To lift the **depression** cloud away.
Used for **major depression**, that heavy load,
Sometimes for **anxiety**, off-label mode.
It **stabilizes mood** with a steady hand,
Though it takes **weeks** to truly stand.

Side effects nurses should know:
Nausea, **dry mouth**, **fatigue**, or **slow flow**.
Sexual dysfunction, **insomnia**, too,
And **sweating** or **tremor** may come through.
There's a risk of **QT prolongation**,
Especially in **higher concentration**.
So monitor with an **EKG**,
If the patient's at risk—cardiology.

Yes, there's a **Black Box Warning** to heed:
Suicidal thoughts may rise with speed—

Especially in youth, so monitor close,

Watch for **agitation**, **mood swings**, morose.

Don't mix with **MAOIs**—a dangerous pair,

Serotonin syndrome could soon flare.

Also caution with **St. John's Wort**,

And other **serotonergic support**.

Before you give, **assess for mood**,

And **thoughts of harm**—be patient and shrewd.

Watch for signs of **mania's spark**,

If the patient has **bipolar** in the dark.

Teach to **take it daily, same time each day**,

And that relief may be **weeks away**.

Tell them not to stop it cold—

Withdrawal symptoms can take hold.

So **Citalopram** brings balance and peace,

But nurses must guide the proper release.

With careful eyes and patient grace,

We help the healing fall in place.

Clonazepam (Klonopin)

Benzodiazepine

A **benzodiazepine**, calm and deep,
It slows the brain and helps with sleep.
Enhances GABA in the nervous track,
So **seizures, panic**, and **tension** pull back.
Used for **seizure disorders, panic attacks**,
And **anxiety** that quietly stacks.
Sometimes off-label for **muscle spasm** pain,
It calms the mind and soothes the strain.

But be aware of side effects:
Drowsiness, dizziness, and slow reflex.
Fatigue, depression, or **confusion's** call,
And **respiratory depression**, worst of all.
There's a **Black Box Warning** you must cite:
Combined with opioids, it dims the light.
Can cause **coma, death**, and **slowed breath**,
So monitor closely to prevent a death.

It's a **Schedule IV controlled drug**,
With **tolerance, dependence**, and **withdrawal** tug.

Stopping it fast? You'll risk a **seizure**,
So **taper slowly**, by doctor procedure.
Avoid with **alcohol** or other **CNS meds**,
That **sedation combo** can mess with heads.
Also caution with **valproate**,
It can raise **levels**—not so great.

Before you give, **assess their mood**,
Check for **suicidal thoughts** that brood.
Track **seizure type, frequency, length,**
And **respiratory status**, pulse and strength.
Teach patients to **avoid driving** at first,
Until they know if the sedative's cursed.
Tell them to **take it as prescribed**,
And not to **share** or let misuse slide.

So **Clonazepam** brings stillness and ease,
But nurses must watch—no room to freeze.
With education, monitoring, and care,
You help them breathe and stay aware.

Clonidine (Catapres)

Alpha-2 adrenergic agonist

A **centrally acting alpha-2 agonist** med,
It calms the brain, slows what's sped.
It **reduces sympathetic outflow** wide,
So **BP** drops and vessels glide.
Used for **hypertension**, **ADHD**, too,
And **withdrawal symptoms**—yes, that's true.
Sometimes for **hot flashes**, **pain**, and more,
It's versatile at calming the core.

But it's not free from side effects:
Drowsiness, **dry mouth**, and **dizzy reflex**.
Bradycardia, **hypotension**, may arise,
And **rebound hypertension** is the biggest surprise.
There's a **Black Box Warning** you must recall:
Don't stop abruptly—that's the fall.
Severe spikes in BP can occur,
So **taper slowly** to reassure.

Before you give, **check BP and heart**,
If **bradycardic**, you may need to part.

Also assess for **mental state**,

Depression can worsen at a concerning rate.

Caution with other **CNS depressants** in mix,

Like **benzos**, **alcohol**, or **opioid** picks

Beta-blockers used with it? Be wise—

Withdraw **clonidine first** to avoid a surprise.

Teach to take it **at bedtime**, slow,

To lessen **daytime drowsy flow**.

Tell them to **rise slowly**, prevent the fall,

And keep **patches** stuck where they won't stall.

Rotate **patch sites**, clean and dry,

And never cut them—just apply.

Tell them **don't skip** or they might spike,

And to **carry a dose** if they're on a long hike.

So **Clonidine** brings pressure down with care,

But nurses must **monitor**, **teach**, and **prepare**.

With guidance strong and education clear,

This med helps calm what we all fear

Clopidogrel (Plavix)

Antiplatelet agent

An **antiplatelet agent**, strong and sleek,
It keeps **clots** from forming in arteries weak.
It **inhibits ADP binding**, that's the key,
So **platelets can't clump**, staying clot-free.
Used to prevent **MI**, **stroke**, and **PAD**,
And after **stents**, it's part of the spree.
It's often paired with **aspirin**, too,
For **dual therapy** when clots could brew.

But with the power to stop a clot,
Comes **bleeding risk**—like it or not.
Watch for **bruising, nosebleeds, GI pain,**
And **bleeding gums** that might remain.
There's a **Black Box Warning** to discuss—
Some people can't **metabolize** it like us.
If you're a **CYP2C19 poor metabolizer**,
The drug may fail as a clot neutralizer.

Before you give, **check for bleeds,**
History of ulcers or **surgery needs**.

Hold it before **surgery or dental work**,

And **monitor CBC**—don't let labs shirk.

It interacts with drugs that **inhibit the liver**,

Like **omeprazole**, which makes its strength wither.

Avoid with **NSAIDs, anticoagulants** too,

Or the **bleeding risk** might come right through.

Teach patients to **report signs of blood**,

Like **black stools, pink urine**, or a sudden flood.

Tell them not to **stop on their own**,

Unless the provider says it's known.

Take **once daily**, with or without food,

Consistency keeps the therapy good.

And remind them that **falls or cuts** might bleed,

So caution is something they really need.

So **Clopidogrel** guards the flow inside,

But **nurses must teach and wisely guide**.

With bleeding risk and platelets tamed,

We help prevent strokes—**lives reclaimed**.

Cyclobenzaprine (Flexeril)

Muscle relaxant

A **muscle relaxant**, central in style,
It helps with **spasms** that cramp and rile.
Acts on the **brainstem**, not the muscle itself,
To calm the tension and restore some health.
Used for **acute muscle pain**, short-term flair,
Like **injuries**, **strains**, and **tightness** there.
Often given with **rest** and **therapy**,
For muscles locked in misery.

But side effects can come in kind:
Drowsiness, **dizziness**, and a **foggy mind**.
Dry mouth, **fatigue**, or even **blurred sight**,
And **constipation** might also bite.
It acts like a **TCA**, so keep in mind,
Its structure and side effects are similarly aligned.
Serotonin syndrome is rare but real,
Especially if mixed with drugs that deal.

No **Black Box Warning**, but still take care,
In **elderly patients**, go slow and beware.

It may worsen **glaucoma**, or **heart blocks** may rise,

So avoid in patients with **cardiac compromise**.

Avoid with **MAOIs**—that's a must,

A **hypertensive crisis** could break your trust.

Caution with **alcohol**, **CNS depressants**, too,

They **amplify sedation** and safety undo.

Before you give, **assess for pain**,

Muscle tone, and what they strain.

Check **mental status**, **fall risk**, too—

Especially if they're **elderly** or new.

Teach to avoid **driving** at first,

Until they know if drowsy is worst.

Tell them this med is **not long-term**,

And **taper if needed**—no crash and burn.

So **Cyclobenzaprine** gives relief with rest,

But nurses must guide for use that's best.

A short-term fix with CNS grace,

Helping tight muscles find their place.

Diclofenac (Voltaren)
NSAID

A strong **NSAID**, it fights with pride,
Pain, **inflammation**, it pushes aside.
It **inhibits COX-1 and COX-2** enzymes tight,
Blocking **prostaglandins** that trigger the fight.
Used for **arthritis**, both **osteo** and **RA**,
Ankylosing spondylitis and **pain** in the day.
Migraines, **dysmenorrhea**, **post-op pain** too,
And it comes in forms from **gel to chew**.

But side effects? They're part of the deal:
GI upset, **ulcers**, **bleeds** that are real.
Headache, dizziness, elevated BP,
And **renal toxicity** is something to see.
There's a **Black Box Warning** you must know:
For **GI bleeding** and **CV risk** flow.
MI, stroke—especially long term,
So monitor closely and confirm.

Also beware of **hepatic strain**,
Check **AST**, **ALT**, again and again.

Kidney function? Don't forget that part—
Watch **BUN** and **creatinine** from the start.
Avoid with other **NSAIDs**, and **blood thinners**, too,
The **bleed risk rises**, that much is true.
Be careful with **ACE inhibitors**, or **diuretics** with name—
They may reduce renal flow and worsen the game.

Teach patients to **take with food or milk**,
To protect the gut like a satin silk.
Tell them to report **bloody stools**,
Or **abdominal pain** that breaks the rules.
The **topical form**? Wash hands after apply,
Avoid **broken skin** and **sunlight's eye**.
For **oral**, swallow whole—no crush or break,
And don't **double dose** for safety's sake.

So **Diclofenac** relieves with might,
But nurses guide to keep it right.
With labs, teaching, and care combined,
We ease the pain and protect the mind.

Diltiazem (Cardizem, Tiazac)

Calcium Channel Blocker (Non-dihydropyridine)

A **calcium channel blocker**, smooth and slow,
It **dilates vessels**, lets **blood pressure** go.
Blocks **calcium entry** in the heart and tone,
To **slow conduction** and **lower pressure** shown.

Used for **hypertension**, **angina pain**,
And **atrial fibrillation** to steady the strain.
Also helps with **SVT** (a fast-paced race),
It brings the **heart rate** to a safer place.

Side effects may still appear:
Bradycardia, **hypotension**, gear.
Dizziness, headache, peripheral swell,
Constipation and **flushing** may as well.

Check **BP** and **apical pulse** before,
If it's under **60**, don't ignore.
Also check for **heart block signs**,
AV node delays in certain lines.

No **Black Box Warning**, but use with care—
In **CHF**, it can worsen the wear.
And with **beta-blockers**, watch the tone,
Can **drop heart rate** or **conduction zone**.

It interacts with **digoxin**, too,
Increasing **dig levels** out of the blue.
Also **CYP3A4 inhibitors** raise its effect,
So monitor labs and what you expect.

Teach patients to **rise slowly** from the bed,
Orthostatic drops may mess with their head.
Take **consistently**, don't skip around,
And **no grapefruit juice** should be found.

So **Diltiazem** calms the heart's wild beat,
Relieves the pressure, makes pulses neat.
With nursing eyes and teaching right,
This med can help both **day and night**.

Doxycycline (Vibramycin)

Tetracycline antibiotic

A **tetracycline antibiotic**, broad and wide,
It stops the bugs from growing inside.
It **binds the 30S ribosomal site**,
And blocks **protein synthesis** outright.
Used for **acne, STIs, respiratory flares**,
Lyme disease, malaria, and **tick-borne scares**.
Also treats **Rocky Mountain spotted fever**,
And **chlamydia** infections—clever, clever.

But side effects still may arise:
Photosensitivity under sunny skies.
Nausea, vomiting, and **diarrhea**, too,
And **esophagitis** if it sticks in you
Don't give it with **milk** or **antacids near**,
They bind the drug and make it unclear.
Space out those doses if calcium's in play—
Or the med won't work the proper way.

There's **no Black Box Warning**, but take note,
In **pregnancy**, it's not a good vote.

It can **stain baby teeth** and **affect bone**,

So keep it away from the fetal zone.

Avoid in **kids under eight years old**,

It may leave **permanent stains** of yellow bold.

And teach to **take it with water upright**,

To stop **GI pain** and keep things right.

It may interact with **warfarin's might**,

So check **INR** to keep things tight.

And **oral contraceptives** may not hold firm,

So **backup birth control** is the nursing term.

Teach patients to **use sunscreen** strong,

And finish the course—don't string it long.

Take it **with food** if nausea hits,

But avoid dairy in those time splits.

So **Doxycycline** stops bugs in stride,

But nurses must help and gently guide.

With timing, teaching, and safety first,

It beats infections before they burst.

Dulaglutide (Trulicity)

GLP-1 receptor agonist (antidiabetic)

A **GLP-1 receptor agonist**, long-acting and neat,
It helps control **blood sugar**—a diabetes feat.
Mimics incretin, slows **gastric flow**,
Boosts **insulin secretion** when glucose is low.
Used for **Type 2 diabetes**, steady and strong,
Helps with **A1C reduction** all week long.
Also brings **weight loss**—a helpful perk,
But it's **not for Type 1**—won't work.

Given by **weekly injection**, subQ style,
It keeps sugar low in a lasting file.
Common sites? **Thigh, abdomen, arm**—
Rotate spots to avoid injection harm.
Watch for **nausea, vomiting, GI pain,**
Diarrhea, fatigue, and **loss of gain.**
Pancreatitis can occur, though rare,
So report **severe belly pain** with care.

There's a **Black Box Warning** loud and clear:
Thyroid C-cell tumors—a rare fear.

Avoid if there's a **family thyroid history**,

Like **MEN2** or **medullary mystery**.

Before you give it, **check blood glucose**,

And assess for **GI issues** that may impose.

Use caution with **renal disease**—

Nausea and dehydration can disrupt ease.

It may interact with **insulin** or **secretagogues**,

So monitor closely for **hypoglycemic logs**.

Slows the **GI tract**, so meds may absorb late—

Be mindful when **timing** other meds on their plate.

Teach patients to store it **cold, not froze**,

And **take it out early** before the dose.

Instruct on **pen use**, **site rotation**,

And signs of **pancreas inflammation**.

So **Dulaglutide** keeps sugar in line,

But nurses must teach and monitor time.

With **weekly care**, and **labs to track**,

It helps bring Type 2 diabetes back.

Duloxetine (Cymbalta)

SNRI antidepressant

An **SNRI**, dual-action and wise,
It lifts low mood and quiets the cries.
Blocks **serotonin** and **norepinephrine** reuptake,
To help the nerves and spirit awake.
Used for **depression** and **anxiety's grip**,
And **nerve pain** that makes life slip.
Also treats **fibromyalgia, diabetic pain,**
And **chronic musculoskeletal strain**.

But side effects may still appear:
Nausea, dry mouth, sweating, and **fear.**
Fatigue, dizziness, and **appetite loss,**
And **insomnia** may come across.
There's a **Black Box Warning** you must teach—
Suicidal thoughts may rise or breach.
Especially in **youth and young adults,**
So **monitor mood** and any results.

Can cause **serotonin syndrome** when combined,
With other **serotonergic meds** aligned.

Agitation, **tremor**, and **fever's** cue—
If those show up, it's time to review
Watch the **liver** if damage is known,
ALT, **AST** should be shown.
Avoid with **alcohol**, it stresses more,
And **hepatic failure** might be in store.

Also watch for **hypertension** raise,
Especially in early treatment days.
It may **worsen glaucoma** too,
So **eye pressure checks** might be due.
Teach patients it takes a **few weeks to act**,
Don't stop cold—**taper** with care intact.
Take **with or without food**, either way,
And report **mood swings** without delay.

So **Duloxetine** brings calm and light,
For mood and pain, it helps make right.
But nurses must **guide, assess, and teach**,
To keep safe healing within reach.

Empagliflozin (Jardiance)

SGLT2 inhibitor

An **SGLT2 inhibitor**, smart and lean,
It works right in the **kidneys' scene**.
Blocks **glucose reabsorption** from the pee,
So sugar's lost through **urinary spree**.
Used for **Type 2 diabetes**, that's its base,
And **heart failure**—it slows the race.
Helps reduce the **cardiac event toll**,
And protects the **kidneys** on the whole.

Side effects? We watch with care:
UTIs and **yeast infections** are common there.
Dehydration, **hypotension**, may arise,
And **ketoacidosis** in rare surprise.
Watch for signs like **nausea, fatigue**,
Abdominal pain—don't let it intrigue.
Euglycemic DKA is sly,
Glucose isn't high, but they still could die.

Before you give, check **renal labs**,
f **GFR is too low**, you may need to grab

Another med—it won't work below

That **eGFR** line—it's good to know.

No **Black Box Warning** at this stage,

But some risks still make the page:

Fournier's gangrene, though very rare,

Means teach them **hygiene** with thoughtful care.

Interactions? **Diuretics**, for sure,

Can raise the **dehydration score**.

And **insulin combos**—be alert,

They may cause **hypoglycemia** hurt.

Teach to **stay hydrated**, monitor signs,

Of **dizzy spells** or **low sugar lines**.

And remind them to report **burning pee**,

Or **unusual discharge** urgently.

So **Empagliflozin** filters the sweet,

Flushes the sugar right off its feet.

But nurses help to guide the plan—

To heal with knowledge, as only we can.

Ergocalciferol (Vitamin D2)

Vitamin D2 supplement

A form of **Vitamin D**, plant-derived,
Helps keep **bones strong** and **calcium** revived.
It's a **fat-soluble vitamin**, not made by sun,
That helps with absorption when daylight's none.
It boosts **calcium** and **phosphorus** stores,
So **bone growth**, **teeth**, and more restores.
Used in **rickets**, and **osteomalacia's** toll,
And **hypoparathyroidism** takes its role.

Also used when **diet is poor**,
Or **deficiency** is shown for sure.
But it takes time and needs the right dose—
Too much, and side effects may diagnose.
Hypercalcemia can lead the way,
With **nausea**, **vomiting**, and **weakness** in play.
Kidney stones, confusion, or **muscle pain**,
From too much **D** in the bloodstream train.

Before you give, **check labs ahead**—
Calcium, phosphate, vitamin D levels read.

Also monitor **renal function**,

To avoid excess or obstruction

There's **no Black Box Warning**, but still be wise,

With **toxicity risk** that can arise.

Especially when **high doses** are long,

Or if the **kidneys** aren't strong.

Interactions may include:

Thiazide diuretics, in hypercalcemia's feud.

And **anticonvulsants** like **phenytoin**,

Which lower **D** levels slowly in time.

Teach to take with **fat-rich meals**,

To help with **absorption** and better deals.

Avoid **over-supplementation** blends,

Especially if taking multiple ends.

So **Ergocalciferol**, D_2 in name,

Supports the bones and metabolic game.

But with **nursing eyes** and **dosing smart**,

We guard the kidneys and protect the heart.

Escitalopram (Lexapro)

SSRI antidepressant

An **SSRI**, smooth and bright,
It helps bring **depression** into light.
Blocks serotonin reuptake flow,
So mood can lift, and peace can grow.
Used for **MDD** and **GAD**,
To ease the weight and clear the gray.
Sometimes used for **panic** and more,
But always **start low**, then slowly explore.

Side effects can still appear:
Nausea, **headache**, and **drowsiness** near.
Sexual dysfunction, **dry mouth**, **sweat**,
And **insomnia** might be a bet.
It carries a **Black Box Warning** too—
Suicidal thoughts may rise in view.
Especially in **teens and young adults**,
So assess their **mood** and emotional results.

Can cause **serotonin syndrome** if paired
With other meds that make serotonin flared:

MAOIs, triptans, St. John's Wort,
Can send the system out of sort.
No need to check labs on the daily,
But **watch for agitation**, acting strangely.
Teach to **never stop abruptly**,
Or withdrawal may hit them subtly.

Dizziness, zaps, or **nausea** can spin,
So taper slow when coming off in the end.
Avoid with **alcohol** or **CNS slows**,
That can increase sedation's lows.
Teach patients: take it **once each day**,
With or without food—it's okay.
And let them know it takes a **few weeks** in,
Before they really feel the win.

So **Escitalopram**, a steady guide,
To calm the storm and lift the tide.
But nurses must watch, assess, and teach,
To keep recovery within safe reach.

Estradiol (Estrace, Climara, Vivelle-Dot)

Estrogen hormone replacement

A form of **estrogen**, pure and true,
It helps when **hormone levels** dip in you.
Treats **menopause**, with **hot flash heat**,
And **vaginal dryness** it helps defeat.
It aids in **bone loss prevention**, too,
When **osteoporosis** starts to break through.
Sometimes used in **hormone therapy**,
For **transgender care** or **ovarian atrophy**.

But risks are real and must be known,
With **thromboembolic events** that have been shown.
Can cause **stroke**, **DVT**, or **PE**,
So nurses assess and monitor carefully
It carries a **Black Box Warning** bright:
Endometrial cancer—keep it in sight.
Also **breast cancer**, **heart disease** rise,
Especially in **long-term use** or higher size.

Side effects include **nausea, bloat,** and **breast pain,**

Mood swings, headache, and **spotting** may remain.

Weight changes, fluid retention, and **cramps,**

Sometimes even **vision** gets a little damp.

Avoid in pregnancy, Category X,

And watch for **liver dysfunction** or **breast exam checks.**

Also avoid with **undiagnosed bleeding,**

Or **estrogen-sensitive tumors** intervening.

Interacts with **rifampin, phenytoin,** and more,

And **smoking** increases **clot risk** galore.

Caution with **thyroid meds** and **insulin use,**

As hormone changes may shake them loose.

Teach patients to use **as directed each time,**

Be it **pill, patch,** or **gel in a line.**

Rotate patch sites, avoid **heat or sun,**

And report any **leg pain** or **chest pain** that's begun.

So **Estradiol** brings balance back,

When **estrogen dips** and symptoms stack.

But nurses must guide, assess with care,

To manage the risk that comes with repair.

Ethinyl Estradiol/Norethindrone (Loestrin, etc.)

Combined hormonal contraceptive

A **combined oral contraceptive**, tried and true,
With **estrogen** and **progestin** working for you.
Suppresses ovulation, thins the **uterine line**,
And thickens **cervical mucus** to block the sign.
Used for **birth control**, and that's not all—
Helps regulate **periods**, makes flow small.
Also treats **acne**, **PMS**, and **PCOS** flare,
Balancing hormones with careful care.

Side effects? Oh yes, they can show:
Nausea, **breast tenderness**, and **spotting flow**.
Mood swings, **bloating**, and **weight shifts**,
And sometimes **libido** takes little dips.
But here comes the **Black Box Warning** sound—
Especially if **smoking** and **over 35** are found.
Thromboembolic risk—stroke, PE, DVT,
So nurses must assess thoroughly.

Don't use it with **migraines with aura** in view,

Or **liver disease**, or **BP too high, too.**

Also contraindicated in **estrogen cancers**,

So **patient history** holds key answers.

Interacts with **rifampin, anticonvulsants**, and more,

May weaken the pill—**backup birth control** is core.

Antibiotics? A debate still remains,

But **educate anyway**, just to explain.

Teach to take it **same time every day**,

And if **missed**, know what the **instructions** say.

Three weeks on, then **one week off** to bleed,

Or sometimes **extended cycles** meet the need.

Watch for signs of **ACHES**—a big red flag:

Abdominal pain, Chest pain, or **Headache** nag.

Eye problems, Swelling, or **leg pain** odd—

Could signal a **clot**, and that's no facade.

So **Ethinyl Estradiol/Norethindrone**

Keeps cycles calm and eggs alone.

But nurses must **teach, assess,** and **guide**,

To keep the risks on the safer side.

Ethinyl Estradiol/Norgestimate (Ortho Tri-Cyclen, etc.)

Combined hormonal contraceptive

A **combo birth control**, hormone-designed,
With **estrogen** and **progestin** combined.
It **prevents ovulation**, keeps cycles tame,
And thickens **mucus** to block sperm's game
Used for **contraception**, **acne control**,
And to help **periods** stay on a roll.
Treats **PMS**, **cycle pain**, and more,
A popular pill with many a score.

Side effects are common to see:
Nausea, **headache**, and **breast tenderness** be.
Mood swings, **spotting**, and **weight that shifts**,
Sometimes **libido** quietly drifts.
But here's the **Black Box Warning**, loud and clear—
Smokers over 35 should steer clear.
Blood clots, **stroke**, **DVT**, or **MI**,
These risks increase and amplify.

Don't use with **high BP** uncontrolled,

Or **estrogen-based cancer** in a story told.

Also avoid with **liver disease**,

And **migraine with aura**—stop it, please.

Interactions are key to know:

Anticonvulsants, **rifampin**, can steal the show.

Antibiotics? A gray zone still,

But best to **use backup** with any new pill.

Teach to take it at the **same time each day**,

To **prevent pregnancy** and keep signs at bay.

Missing pills? Review the **"what to do"**,

Whether it's one or two—or even a few.

Watch for the acronym **ACHES** with care:

Abdominal pain, **Chest pain**, **Headaches** rare,

Eye changes, **Swelling** or **leg pain** too—

Could be a **clot**, so follow through.

So **Ethinyl Estradiol/Norgestimate**

Keeps things on track and regulates.

But nurses must guide with facts that stick,

To keep this birth control safe and quick.

Ezetimibe (Zetia)

Cholesterol Absorption Inhibitor

A lipid-lowering agent, quite refined,
Blocks cholesterol where intestines bind.
Cell cycle-nonspecific, it works with grace,
Reducing fats that the gut might embrace.
Prescribed alone or with statins too,
For **hyperlipidemia**, it helps you through.
Familial high cholesterol is on the list,
A non-statin ally you won't want to miss.

Side effects are mild but worth the call—
Fatigue, joint pain, and sometimes gall.
Rare but real are **angioedema** flares,
And **hepatitis** risk, so monitor with care.
Check LFTs before you start,
And during therapy, play the smart part.
Creatine kinase if muscles ache,
To rule out rhabdo for safety's sake.

Before the med, a lipid panel's due,
During and after, recheck values too.

Patient should follow a **low-fat diet**,
And take it **daily**—please don't fight it!
Take **without regard to meals**, that's fine,
But **space from bile acid sequestrants in time**.
(Wait two hours after or four hours before—
This helps absorption, and opens the door.)

If **crushing** is needed, it can be done,
But mix with water and don't make it fun.
Store it in **cool, dry** places tight,
Away from moisture and direct light.
Wear gloves if needed for safety zones,
Though oral pills don't leach through bones.
But handle with care and know the plan—
Especially if prepping for a scan.

No major CYP action, so few drug wars,
But **avoid with fibrates**—they may cause sores.
And in combo with statins, risk might rise—
So monitor **liver and muscle** for warning signs.

Famotidine (Pepcid)

H2 Receptor Antagonist

It calms the stomach's acid tide,
Blocks H2 histamine on the gastric side.
Reduces secretions that love to burn,
Giving ulcers and GERD a helpful turn.

Cell cycle-nonspecific, it's steady and strong,
Works day or night to right what's wrong.
Used for **GERD, ulcers, Zollinger-Ellison too**,
And stress ulcer prophylaxis in ICU.

Side effects aren't common, but keep in mind—
Headache, dizziness, and a confused kind.
Especially in elders, it might cause delay,
In mental clarity or what they say.

Rare but real is **thrombocytopenia**,
So monitor CBC if they feel anemia.
Can raise **creatinine** without true decline,
So **kidney labs** should look just fine.

Before you give, **check renal function** tight,
A **dose reduction** may be just right.
No need for meals, but if they do,
It won't harm—it's safe to chew.

It comes in oral, IV form as well,
Push **IV over 2 minutes**—don't make cells yell!
If giving by drip, go slow and wise,
Dilute and infuse, no rapid surprise.

No special gloves, but always clean hands,
Prep with care and follow your plans.
Watch for IV **infiltration** signs,
Redness, pain—draw those lines.

With **antacids**, it can still be used,
But **don't give with sucralfate**—it gets confused.
Space them **at least 2 hours apart**,
To give both meds a proper start.

Fenofibrate (Tricor)

Fibric Acid Derivative (Fibrate Class)

It lowers fats, but not through the gut,
It boosts lipase so **triglycerides** get cut.
A **PPAR-alpha activator**, sleek and lean,
Clears blood of lipids and keeps vessels clean.

Cell cycle-nonspecific, but sharp and wise,
It's used when **triglycerides start to rise**.
For **mixed dyslipidemia** or high fat alone,
And in combo with statins—though not overblown.

Side effects may include **GI distress**,
Like nausea, pain, and gas, no less.
Watch for **muscle pain or weakness flair**,
Could be **rhabdo**—check with care.

Liver enzymes may climb too high,
So monitor **AST, ALT** and ask why.
Check **renal function** before you start,
Especially in elders—play the smart part.

Start with **labs**—a **lipid panel** clean,
Then repeat at **4–8 weeks** to see the scene.
LFTs baseline and **periodically after**,
And **CK** if muscle pain causes chatter.

Take it **with food**, that's how it's done,
Boosts absorption for everyone.
Capsule form—don't crush or split,
Just swallow whole for a better fit.

Handle like any oral med,
No PPE unless your policy said.
Store in a **cool, dry place** with care,
Keep the bottle closed, no open air.

With **statins**, watch for muscle doom,
And **anticoagulants**—they increase the room.
So adjust **warfarin dose** with INR in sight,
To avoid a bleed that's not polite.

Finasteride (Proscar, Propecia)

5-Alpha Reductase Inhibitor

It shrinks the **prostate**, calms the stream,
And boosts hair growth like a dream.
By **blocking DHT**, it makes its stand—
That's **dihydrotestosterone** it bans firsthand.
Cell cycle-nonspecific, slow but true,
Used for **BPH** and **baldness too**.
Proscar for **prostates**, Propecia for **hair**,
But both require patient care.

Side effects? They're not a ton,
But **erectile dysfunction** may come.
Decreased **libido**, mood that dips,
And **gynecomastia** (male breast tips).
Watch for signs of **depression** deep,
And **suicidal thoughts** that sometimes creep.
No urgent labs for all who try,
But **PSA levels** could go awry.

Before you give, check **PSA baseline**,
Then monitor levels as they decline.

Because finasteride will cut it in half,

So **doubling the PSA** gives the real graph.

Take with or without food, it's fine,

But **daily dosing** must align.

Warn patients: **effects take months to show**,

Don't stop early—results are slow.

Pregnant women, beware this pill!

Don't touch—**it's teratogenic still**.

Affects male fetuses in the womb,

So **gloves for crushed tablets**—assume!

No blood donation for **6 months after**,

To protect unborn sons from this disaster.

Handle with care, store safe and tight,

In a cool, dry place, out of the light.

It doesn't mix with many meds,

But **saw palmetto**—watch those threads.

That herb can **amplify effects**,

So always ask what one selects.

Fluoxetine (Prozac)
Selective Serotonin Reuptake Inhibitor (SSRI)

It lifts the fog and fights despair,
Boosts **serotonin** floating there.
Blocks its reuptake, leaves more behind—
To soothe the **depressed and anxious mind**.
Though **cell cycle-nonspecific** it be,
It acts on mood **neurochemistry**.
Used for **MDD, OCD**, and more,
Bulimia, panic, and even **PMDD's war**.

Side effects come, so stay alert—
GI upset, insomnia, or head that hurts.
Can cause **sexual dysfunction**, too,
And **weight gain or loss**—for just a few.
Rare but deadly: **serotonin storm**,
Agitation, fever—**not the norm**.
Tremor, twitching, mental change—
Call the doctor—it's getting strange.

Start with **mental health assessment**, clean,
Check for **suicidal thoughts** unseen.

Monitor for **mood swings, sleep, and weight**,

And **labs** if long-term—**LFTs** relate.

Give it **in the morning**—it can excite,

Though some may need it **at night**.

With or without food, both are okay,

Just be **consistent**—same time each day.

Taper slowly if ending the ride,

Stopping too fast can **shock the mind**.

No need for gloves, but wash with care,

If crushing's needed—mix with flair.

Black Box Warning: suicide risk may climb,

Especially in teens over time.

So educate well and stay in touch,

Frequent check-ins matter much.

No MAOIs within 14 days,

Or **serotonin syndrome** lights ablaze.

And **watch with NSAIDs** or those that thin—

Bleeding risk may creep within.

Fluticasone (Flonase, Flovent)

Corticosteroid – Anti-Inflammatory Agent

A **steroid spray** or **inhaled mist**,
Reduces swelling where symptoms persist.
It tames the fire of **inflammation**,
In lungs or nose—it brings salvation.
Cell cycle-nonspecific, yet strong and clear,
It **reduces histamines** and calms what's near.
Used for **asthma, COPD, rhinitis too**,
And **seasonal allergies** bothering you.

Side effects are mostly mild,
But worth a watch in every child:
Throat irritation, hoarse voice tone,
Nasal burning if used alone.
Can cause **oral thrush**—that yeast might bloom,
So **rinse the mouth** to clear the room.
In rare events, **adrenal suppression**,
So monitor growth in each progression.

Peak flow, lung sounds, and **O_2 stats**,
Track how the breathing slowly adapts.

For nasal use, **inspect the nose**,

Check for **ulcers, bleeding**, or tissue that grows.

Before the dose, they should blow their nose,

Or for inhalers, shake before those flows.

Take **bronchodilator first**, then wait,

Fluticasone follows—that's the gate.

Rinse the mouth to keep thrush away,

Clean the device at end of day.

Don't stop abruptly—**taper with care**,

Systemic steroids may still be there.

Handle with gloves if policy says,

Though often not needed in modern ways.

But treat it like any med with respect,

And teach them well what to expect.

No wild drug wars, but take this hint:

Other steroids can cause a sprint.

Additive effects can **suppress the axis**,

So note the signs—avoid the crisis.

Fluticasone/Salmeterol (Advair Diskus)

Inhaled Corticosteroid + Long-Acting Beta-2 Agonist

A **combo drug**, two powers unite—
One calms **inflammation**, one brings **breath back to light**.
Fluticasone soothes with steroid grace,
While **Salmeterol** opens the airway space.
Cell cycle-nonspecific, but key in its might,
It keeps **asthma** and **COPD** patients breathing right.
It's a **maintenance med**, not for rescue breath,
So don't grab it first in a **wheezing** death.

Side effects can still appear,
Thrush, **headache**, **tremor**, maybe fear.
Palpitations, **nervousness**, or **voice that's hoarse**,
Even **high BP** in some, of course.
Teach patients well, **rinse mouth each time**,
To keep **oral candidiasis** from its climb.
Monitor lungs and **heart rate**, too—
Check **peak flow readings** for what they do.

Before they take it, have them prep:

Exhale fully, then take a deep step.

Inhale quick and deep, then hold their breath,

For **10 seconds max**, like a mindful stretch.

No need to **shake** this Diskus dry,

Just slide, inhale, and let time fly.

Bronchodilator still goes first, then wait,

Five minutes later, Advair's great.

Gloves not needed, but storage is smart—

Dry and room temp, keep it apart.

No wet devices, don't wash or soak,

A simple wipe keeps it bespoke.

Avoid with other long-acting B2s,

Too much stimulation might blow a fuse.

Watch with **CYP3A4 inhibitors**, too—

They **boost steroid levels**, make side effects new.

Black Box Warning: don't use alone

The **LABA** part must have a **steroid tone**.

That's why they're paired in this Diskus blend—

To keep inflammation and spasms at end.

Folic Acid (Vitamin B9)

Water-Soluble Vitamin – Hematinic Agent

It builds your blood and grows your brain,
Supports your cells and eases strain.
DNA synthesis is its core game,
And **RBC formation** is its claim to fame.

Though **cell cycle-nonspecific**, it plays a role,
In every phase that makes you whole.
Used for **deficiency**, often in **pregnancy**,
And for **megaloblastic anemia's urgency**.

Neural tube defects—it helps prevent,
So **prenatal use** is time well spent.
Also given with **methotrexate**,
To guard the cells while it sedates.

Side effects are rare and small,
But allergic **rash** can still befall.
Bronchospasm or **itchy skin**,
Though mostly safe when taken in.

Check **folate levels** at the start,
And monitor **CBC** to do your part.
In anemia, track **H&H**—
Ensure the red cell count comes back.

No prep needed—**just take it oral**,
Or **IM, IV**, if it's more formal.
With or without food, both are okay,
Just take it daily—don't delay.

If giving **IV**, go slow and smooth,
Dilute it down and let it soothe.
No special gloves for this routine,
But clean technique keeps the site pristine.

It plays nice with most meds you'll find,
But **methotrexate and sulfa** come to mind.
Phenytoin, too, may clash a bit—
Folate can lower seizure med's hit.

Furosemide (Lasix)

Loop Diuretic – Antihypertensive Agent

It works in the **loop of Henle's bend**,
To pull off fluid and help hearts mend.
It blocks **Na⁺ and Cl⁻ reabsorption**, too,
So water follows, flushing through.
Cell cycle-nonspecific, but bold,
Used when **edema** or **BP's uncontrolled**.
For **CHF, renal disease**, and more,
It opens up that **fluid-clogged door**.

Side effects—you'll want to know:
Hypokalemia steals the show.
Also watch for **low sodium**, **mag**,
And **hypotension**—don't let them sag.
Ototoxicity is rare but real,
So **push it slow**—that's the deal.
It may raise **uric acid, glucose**, too,
So diabetics might need something new.

Check **K⁺ and electrolytes** before,
Along with **BUN, creatinine score**.

Watch **daily weights, I&Os**,

And note how well the urine flows.

Give in the morning, not at night,

To avoid those bathroom flights.

If IV, **no faster than 20mg/min**,

To protect their hearing from within.

Monitor BP, it may go low,

And **orthostatic** symptoms may show.

Encourage potassium-rich food intake—

Like bananas, spinach, or even a shake.

Handle with care, but gloves not a must,

Just follow policies you trust.

Store it safe from heat and light,

Keep it dry and sealed up tight.

Avoid with digoxin unless K⁺ is stable,

Or **toxicity** may join the table.

And with **NSAIDs**, it may not work—

They blunt its power and let fluid lurk.

Gabapentin (Neurontin)

Anticonvulsant – Neuropathic Pain Agent

It's not a benzo, not a narcotic,
But calms the nerves when they get chaotic.
Modulates calcium in CNS zones,
And **mimics GABA**, though it stands alone.

Cell cycle-nonspecific, slow and chill,
Prescribed for **seizures** or **nerve pain's will**.
Postherpetic neuralgia, fibro flare,
And off-label for **anxiety** or **hot flash care**.

Side effects that you may find—
Drowsiness, dizziness, a foggy mind.
Ataxia, fatigue, and **edema feet**,
So fall precautions make it neat.

Taper slow—**don't quit too fast**,
Or **seizures, rebound** pain may last.
Suicidal thoughts may creep in view,
So monitor mood and feelings too.

Check **renal labs** before you go,
Since it's cleared by kidneys slow.
Dose may change if **function's poor**,
So creatinine tells what's in store.

Take it **with or without food**,
But **don't crush extended-release**, dude.
Divide the doses throughout the day,
To keep those levels smooth and stay.

Don't drive till they know how they react,
It hits the brain—**be mindful of that**.
Store it in a **cool, dry place**,
Away from kids and pet's embrace.

Watch if combined with other meds,
Especially **CNS depressant threads**.
Opioids, benzos, alcohol too—
Can cause sedation, fall risk in view.

Glimepiride (Amaryl)

Sulfonylurea – Oral Hypoglycemic Agent

It helps the **pancreas secrete more juice**,
That **insulin** flow gets a power boost.
By **stimulating beta cells** to act,
It keeps blood sugar on the right track.
Cell cycle-nonspecific, but plays a role,
In managing **Type 2 diabetes control**.
Used when **diet and exercise alone**
Can't bring that **A1C** back home.

Side effects to keep in view—
Hypoglycemia is the big one, too!
May also cause **weight to rise**,
And **nausea**, **rash**, or **sun-sensitive eyes**.
Rare but serious—**aplastic lines**,
Like **anemia, low platelets**, or **WBC signs**.
So monitor **CBC** if symptoms appear,
Like bruising, bleeding, or fever near.

Check **blood glucose** before each dose,
And monitor trends—keep them close.

Track their **HbA1c** every few,
To see if long-term goals are true.
Take it **with breakfast**, once a day,
Helps **reduce GI upset** that way.
If they skip a meal—**skip the pill**,
Or hypoglycemia might make them ill.

No crushing tablets—just swallow whole,
And teach them how to check glucose control.
Watch for signs of sugar too low—
Sweating, **shaking**, or **mental fog slow**.
Gloves aren't needed for handling this,
Just follow protocol—don't miss.
Store in a **cool and dry** location,
Tightly capped with no vibration.

Avoid with alcohol—that mix is rough,
It can cause **flushing** or drops that're tough.
Caution with **beta-blockers** too—
They can **mask low sugar's early clue**.

Glipizide (Glucotrol)

Sulfonylurea – Oral Hypoglycemic Agent

It's a **pancreas pusher**, insulin boost,
Helps those **beta cells** cut sugar loose.
By binding channels that close the gate,
It triggers **insulin release**—first-rate!
Cell cycle-nonspecific, still key,
Treats **Type 2 diabetes** effectively.
When **diet and exercise** just won't do,
This med can help to balance you.

Side effects? Let's name a few:
Hypoglycemia—the biggest cue.
Also may cause **weight to gain**,
Or **nausea, headache, stomach pain**.
Photosensitivity may appear,
So sunscreen use should be clear.
Rarely **blood dyscrasias** sneak—
So **CBC** if patients feel weak.

Check blood glucose pre-dose each day,
And track that **A1C** on the way.

Watch for signs of sugar that's low:

Sweaty, shaky, slow to know.

Take it **30 minutes before a meal**,

So the **pancreas pumps with every deal**.

Skipping meals? Skip the dose,

So lows don't strike and cause a close.

Extended-release? Don't crush or break—

Let it dissolve at its own pace.

Immediate-release? That's fine to chew,

But follow prescriber instructions true.

No gloves required, just handle clean,

Store at **room temp**, cool and lean.

Label clear, and patient taught—

So dosing errors won't be caught.

Alcohol can worsen low BG,

So teach them: no shots, wine, or spree.

Beta-blockers, too, can **mask the signs**,

So check the sugar—even if they feel fine.

Hydrochlorothiazide (Microzide)

Thiazide Diuretic – Antihypertensive Agent

It works down in the **distal tubule zone**,
Where **sodium and chloride** would call home.
It blocks their reabsorption—makes water go,
So **BP drops** and **urine flows**.

Though **cell cycle-nonspecific**, it plays its part,
In easing the pressure on a weary heart.
Used for **hypertension**, **edema**, too—
From **CHF**, or **liver** backup in view.

Side effects? Let's name the big:
Hypokalemia—that's no gig.
Also **low sodium**, **high calcium**, and **uric acid rise**,
So **gout** and **kidney stones** may surprise.

May also raise **glucose** in some,
So **diabetics** need to stay on the run.
Dizziness, **headache**, and **photosensitivity**,
Can come with long-term activity.

Monitor **electrolytes**, especially K⁺,
And **BUN/creatinine** every so many days.
Track **daily weights**, and **I&O**,
To gauge how well the fluids flow.

Give it **in the morning**, not near bed,
Or they'll be in the bathroom instead.
Take it with food to **calm the gut**,
And **hydrate well** to keep things shut.

Gloves aren't needed, but storage is right—
Keep it dry and sealed from light.
Teach them about the **sun's bright rays**—
They might burn fast on sunny days.

Watch with **digoxin**, if K⁺ **drops low**,
Toxicity risk begins to grow.
And **lithium levels** may get too high—
So monitor both and tell them why.

Hydrocodone/Acetaminophen (Norco, Vicodin, Lortab)

Opioid Analgesic + Non-Opioid Analgesic (Acting Combo)

A **duo med** for **moderate pain**,
It hits the brain, not just the strain.
Hydrocodone binds to opioid sites,
While **acetaminophen** dulls the spikes.
Cell cycle–nonspecific, strong and fast,
Relief that's meant to **briefly last**.
Used for **post-op, injury,** or **chronic aches**,
But comes with **warnings** for safety's sake.

Side effects—a classic list:
Drowsiness, dizziness, can't be missed.
Nausea, vomiting, constipation, too,
And **respiratory depression**—a real issue.
The **opioid risk** is front and center,
So check **RR**, O_2 sat, and mental enter.
Hold the dose if RR is below 12,
And notify the doc—don't try to delve.

Acetaminophen, the gentler side,
Can still cause **liver damage** if amplified.
So teach: **4,000 mg/day is the ceiling**,
Too much can hurt without much feeling.
Start with **pain scale** before each dose,
And reassess once relief is close.
Vitals, **bowel sounds**, and signs of misuse—
Monitor closely, don't let it confuse.

Give it **with food** to soothe the gut,
And warn: **no booze**—that's a dangerous cut.
No crushing unless it's IR,
Extended-release needs special care.
Store it tight, **double-locked** and neat,
A **Schedule II** drug—diversion's discreet.
Educate on **dependence signs**,
And **wean off slowly** over time.

Avoid with benzos and other CNS downers,
Or risk a visit from ER towners.
Naloxone nearby in case of a fall,
An antidote nurse should recall.

Hydroxyzine (Vistaril, Atarax)

Antihistamine – Anxiolytic, Antiemetic, Sedative

A **first-gen antihistamine** through and through,
With **sedative** and **anti-anxiety** powers too.
It blocks **H1 receptors** in the brain,
Easing **itch, nausea,** and **mental strain**.

Though **cell cycle-nonspecific**, it plays a role,
In calming nerves and gaining control.
Used for **pruritus, allergic flares,**
Anxiety, nausea, even **pre-op care**.

Side effects you're sure to see:
Drowsiness, dry mouth, and **low energy**.
Also **dizziness, blurred sight,** and more—
Anticholinergic effects galore.

Caution with **older adults**, who may
Become **confused** or fall away.
It may **lower seizure threshold**, too,
So know their history through and through.

Vital signs and **LOC** should be checked,
If sedation deepens—redirect.
Monitor for **urinary retention**,
And **bowel status**—give prevention.

Give it **with or without a meal**,
But **IM is deep Z-track**—that's the deal.
Don't give IV—it's not approved,
Only **oral** or **deep IM** is used.

Handle with gloves if policy guides,
But often it's fine—just clean both sides.
Store in a place that's dry and cool,
And label clearly—that's the rule.

Avoid with alcohol, sleep meds, and such,
They'll **amplify drowsy**—a bit too much.
MAOIs and opioids raise concern,
So check their meds at every turn.

Ibuprofen (Advil, Motrin)

NSAID – Nonsteroidal Anti-Inflammatory Drug

It **blocks COX enzymes**, one and two,
To stop the pain from breaking through.
Reduces **fever**, **pain**, and **swelling**,
But has some risks—worth the telling.
Cell cycle-nonspecific, yes indeed,
It meets many a **common need**.
Used for **arthritis, injury, mild to mod pain**,
And **fever** relief in sun or rain.

Side effects—take special note:
GI upset, like **ulcers** or **bloat**.
Can lead to **bleeding** or **kidney decline**,
Especially when used over time.
Also watch for **HTN spikes**,
And **fluid retention** in some types.
May raise **heart attack risk** with length,
So lowest dose, shortest strength.

Check **renal labs** and **BUN/Cr**—
Especially in elders or those with a scar.

CBC too, if bleeding's a fear,

And ask if they've had **black stools** appear.

Give with **food or milk** to coat,

So GI pain won't rock the boat.

For IV form, **infuse it slow**,

Over **30 minutes**, let it flow.

No special handling, but be wise,

Store in a cool place, sealed from skies.

Check for **allergies**—like aspirin kind,

Cross-reactivity's not far behind.

Avoid with **anticoagulants**,

Or **glucocorticoids**—they'll enhance

The **risk for GI bleeding** fast,

So monitor stools till pain has passed.

Pregnancy? Nope—not **third trimester**,

It may shut down that fetal shifter

(**Ductus arteriosus**, to be exact),

So steer clear then—it's a well-known fact.

Insulin Aspart (NovoLog)
Rapid-Acting Insulin Analog

A **rapid-acting insulin**, clear and quick,
It mimics **endogenous insulin's** trick.
It drops blood sugar in a flash,
But peaks too soon—so **eat with your stash**.

It starts to work in **10 to 20**,
Minutes that fly—it doesn't wait any.
Though **cell-cycle phases** don't apply,
Timing with meals is the reason why.

Used for **Type 1** and **Type 2 DM**,
To keep blood sugars calm again.
Given via **pen, pump, or subQ**,
Right before meals—it's the thing to do.

Watch for signs of **hypoglycemia**:
Shaky, sweaty, blurred academia.
Can cause **lipodystrophy** or rash,
Or **weight gain** if you're storing cash.

Be careful—**double-check that pen**,
A **med error here** can do you in.
Don't **mix with glargine**—that's a fact,
Each insulin has its own distinct act.

Monitor **blood glucose** at the start,
Check **A1C** to do your part.
Watch for drops in **potassium**, too—
Hypokalemia can sneak up on you.

Ensure there's **food** on their plate,
Before injecting—don't be late.
Observe them close, assess the signs,
Dizzy, **confused**, or crossing lines.

Inject in **abdomen**, **thigh**, or **arm**,
Rotate sites to prevent harm.
Avoid old bruises, lumps, or skin,
Switch it up to keep health in.

Store **unopened pens** inside the fridge,
But once it's used? You're off that bridge.
Room temp's fine for **28 days**,
But throw it out when it decays.

Be cautious with **beta blockers**, too—
They mask the lows and could fool you.
Corticosteroids raise the score,

So monitor sugars even more.

Insulin Glargine (Lantus, Basaglar)

Long-Acting Insulin Analog

A **long-acting insulin**, slow and neat,
It **mimics basal insulin's beat**.
With **no real peak**, it's steady and flat—
Just one daily dose, and that is that.

It's **cell-cycle neutral**, not tied to a phase,
But maintains control through all your days.
Used for **Type 1** or **Type 2** alone,
Or with short-acting, depending on tone.

Watch for **hypoglycemia** creeping in slow,
It won't come fast—but it can still show.
May cause **weight gain**, **swelling**, or itch,
Or **lipodystrophy** if you don't switch.

Do not mix with other meds in a pen,
It alters the structure—danger again.
Clear solution, but don't confuse,
It's **not for IV or IM** use.

INSULIN GLARGINE (LANTUS, BASAGLAR)

Monitor **blood sugar** and **A1C**,

Check **electrolytes**—especially **K**.

Watch for **low potassium** signs,

Like cramps or weakness down the line.

Give it **once daily**, same time each night,

Preferably **PM** to keep levels right.

Inject **subQ**, not into veins,

And **rotate sites** to avoid the strains.

Prefilled pens or vials on hand,

Store **unopened in fridge**—that's the plan.

Once opened? Keep at **room temp**,

28 days—then time to exempt.

It may interact with **beta blockers**,

Which **mask low sugar's key shockers**.

Steroids and **thiazides** raise blood sugar too,

So monitor closely when those pass through.

Insulin Lispro (Humalog, Admelog)

Rapid-Acting Insulin Analog

A **rapid-acting insulin**, swift to start,
It mimics the **body's insulin part**.
Onset in minutes, peaks in an hour,
So give with food—or risk a power.
No tie to a **cell cycle** here,
But its **fast absorption** is very clear.
Used in **Type 1** and **Type 2** with grace,
To keep blood sugar in its place.

Risk for **hypoglycemia** is real,
Sweating and shaking, a lightheaded feel.
Can also cause **lipodystrophy**,
Or mild **weight gain** over time, you'll see.
Timing is key—give right before meals,
It acts so fast, delay reveals
A danger zone if food's not near—
Always confirm a tray is here.

SubQ route is how it's done,
In **abdomen**, **thigh**, or **upper arm**.

INSULIN LISPRO (HUMALOG, ADMELOG)

Use a **new site** each time you go,
To avoid hard spots or bruises below.
Do not mix in the same syringe
With glargine or detemir—that's a fringe.
Each insulin type has its role and space,
Respect the route, the dose, the pace.

Check **blood glucose** before each dose,
And monitor **A1C** the most.
Watch for **potassium** dropping low—
Hypokalemia is no small show.
Store in the **fridge** until it's used,
Then **28 days** at room temp, not abused.
Keep away from **heat or light**,
And toss it out when it's not right.

It may react with other meds,
Like **steroids**, **diuretics**, or **beta heads**.
These can raise or mask the signs,
So assess your patient's overlapping lines.

Lamotrigine (Lamictal)

Anticonvulsant / Mood Stabilizer

An anticonvulsant, calm and clear,
It keeps **seizures** and **bipolar swings** in gear.
Used in epilepsy and **mood control**,
It **modulates sodium**—that's its role.

It stabilizes **neuronal fire**,
By slowing signals that misfire.
For **tonic-clonic** and **Lennox-Gastaut**,
And in **bipolar depression**, it smooths things out.

But here's the warning: **watch the skin**—
Stevens-Johnson could begin.
Toxic epidermal necrolysis too,
If rash appears, stop—don't push through.

Common side effects? You may find
Dizziness, drowsiness, or fog of mind.
Headache, blurred vision, or **nausea** next,
And sometimes mood swings that leave one vexed.

LAMOTRIGINE (LAMICTAL)

Start this med **low and go slow**,

To prevent the **rash** that's feared, you know.

Doses **must be titrated right**,

Especially if other **AEDs** are in sight.

Monitor for **suicidal thought**,

Especially early, when changes are sought.

Check **liver function**, **CBC**, and skin—

Report all changes, outside or in.

Take with or without a meal,

But take it daily—keep things real.

Don't double dose if one is missed,

Just wait for the next—you get the gist.

Oral tablets, **chewables**, and **dispersible forms**,

Even **XR** for once-daily norms.

Be careful when switching between,

The timing and dosing must be clean.

Interacts with many other meds—

Valproate, in fact, may raise its stead.

While others like **carbamazepine**

Can make lamotrigine less seen.

Pregnancy? It's complex, too—

Risks exist, but seizures do, too.

So weigh it all with OB care,

And always counsel—be aware.

Latanoprost (Xalatan)

Prostaglandin Analog – Antiglaucoma Agent

A **prostaglandin analog**, used in the eye,
To lower **IOP** that's running high.
In **open-angle glaucoma**, it shines,
And for **ocular hypertension**, it realigns.
It works by **increasing outflow** of fluid,
From the **uveoscleral** path—yes, that's how they do it.
Not tied to cell cycles, but timing's tight—
Daily at bedtime is usually right.

Don't be shocked when **eye color may change**,
Iris darkening isn't that strange.
Longer lashes, **lid darkening**, too—
These cosmetic shifts might show through.
Common effects? A **stinging eye**,
Blurred vision, **itching**, maybe dry.
Conjunctival hyperemia's red and sore,
Or **foreign body feeling** you can't ignore.

But the most severe, though rare to find,
Is **macular edema**, especially in kind

With **aphakic patients** or those with lens ops,
So monitor vision if clarity drops.
Before you give, **check contacts are out**—
Wait **15 minutes**—then there's no doubt.
Store in the **fridge** before it's opened,
Then **room temp's fine for 6 weeks** spoken.

One **drop in the evening**, don't overdo,
And **press the lacrimal duct**—that's your cue.
To **prevent systemic absorption**, you see,
And avoid unwanted side effects, possibly.
Don't mix with other drops too close,
Wait 5 minutes between each dose.
And always **wash hands** before you start—
Infection control plays a big part.

May interact with **NSAIDs** or eye meds,
So **check the list** before it's spread.
Report any **vision changes** quick,
Blurred or halos? That's not a trick.

Levothyroxine (Synthroid, Levoxyl, Euthyrox)

Thyroid Hormone Replacement (T4)

A **thyroid hormone**, pure and clean,
It replaces what should have been.
In **hypothyroidism**, it fills the gap,
Giving metabolism its needed snap.

It mimics **T4**, the hormone slow,
Converted to **T3** to make things go.
It binds to receptors across the land,
Controlling growth with a steady hand.

For **Hashimoto's**, goiter, or **post-surgery care**,
Or after **radioactive iodine's** flare.
It treats **cretinism** in kids, too—
Helping their growth and brain come through.

Start **low and go slow**, especially in age,
Or patients with **cardiac history** on stage.
Too much can cause **thyrotoxicity**,

Palpitations, **tremor**, or **anxiety**.

Expect some **weight loss**, that's not rare,
But watch for signs like **feeling too aware**.
Insomnia, **fever**, **sweating**, and more—
Signs of dose being too high at the core.

Take it **first thing**, on an **empty gut**,
With water only—keep the routine shut.
Wait **30 to 60 minutes** before you eat,
Or absorption drops and it's incomplete.

Do not mix with calcium or iron—
They block the drug, and that's no fun.
Antacids too, or fiber bulk,
Can bind the med and make it sulk.

Monitor TSH to guide your path,
Check labs in **6 to 8 weeks'** math.
Too little? Still tired and slow.
Too much? Heart races, symptoms grow.

Teach patients this is **life-long care**,
Missing doses? **Don't you dare**.
It's not a med you **feel right away**,
But stopping it brings symptoms back to stay.

Safe in **pregnancy**, but adjust the dose—

LEVOTHYROXINE (SYNTHROID, LEVOXYL, EUTHYROX)

The need for hormone will often grow most.

Tell the doctor at the first OB scan,

To bump it up and track the plan.

Lisdexamfetamine (Vyvanse)

Central Nervous System Stimulant – Prodrug of Dextroamphetamine

A **CNS stimulant**, slow to begin,
A **prodrug** that's activated from within.
It turns to **dextroamphetamine** with time,
For **ADHD** and **binge eating**—it works just fine.

It **boosts norepinephrine and dopamine**,
Helping focus become more clean.
Improves attention, impulse control,
But misuse risks take a toll.

It's **not tied to a cell cycle frame**,
But timing still plays in the stimulant game.
Take it **early in the morning light**,
Or you'll be **tossing and turning at night**.

Watch for **insomnia, dry mouth**, and **jitter**,
Decreased appetite—a frequent critter.
Increased heart rate, BP climbs,
Even **tics** or **mood swings** at times.

LISDEXAMFETAMINE (VYVANSE)

There's **risk for misuse**, so monitor close,
Especially in teens or those diagnosed
With **substance history** in the past—
This med can be addictive fast.

Assess **baseline vitals** before you start,
BP, **HR**, and **cardiac chart**.
Watch **growth in children**—height and weight,
As stimulants can slow growth rate.

Give it **once daily**, not crushed or chewed,
Capsules can open if child-approved.
Mix powder in **water, yogurt, or juice**,
But take it fast—it's no long-term mousse.

Avoid with **MAOIs**—within **14 days**,
Can cause **hypertensive crisis** in terrifying ways.
Also avoid **acidic foods**,
Which slow absorption and shift its moods.

Monitor behavior, thoughts, and mood,
Watch for **aggression** or attitudes skewed.
Check for **new psychosis**, thoughts that alarm—
Stop the med if there's any harm.

Store in a **safe, locked** place at home,
Controlled **Schedule II**, not left to roam.

Refills require a **new Rx**,

And always follow your **state law checks**.

Lisinopril (Prinivil, Zestril)

ACE Inhibitor – Antihypertensive

An **ACE inhibitor**, tried and true,
It **blocks angiotensin**—part two.
This lowers **BP** and **eases the heart**,
By telling the vessels to stay apart.

Used for **hypertension**, strong and wise,
For **heart failure** and **post-MI** surprise.
It **protects the kidneys** in diabetes,
Slowing damage from nephropathies.

But beware the **cough**, dry and tight,
A side effect that comes at night.
And if the tongue or face does swell?
Angioedema—not so well.

May cause **hypotension**, dizzy and faint,
Especially in those who are weak or ain't
Replenished on salt or volume full—
First-dose drop can be quite dull.

Watch **potassium**, it can rise,

Leading to **hyperkalemia**—no surprise.

Check **renal labs**, like **BUN** and **Cr**,

Especially in those with kidney scar.

Take it **daily**, with or without food,

But same time each day keeps it good.

Avoid **salt substitutes** that sneak in K,

And **NSAIDs** that can lead you astray.

Pregnancy warning: Don't take when with child,

It can harm the fetus—outcomes wild.

Switch to safer meds instead,

Once those two lines are clearly read.

Teach patients signs of **swelling and cough**,

If either appears, the med comes off.

Monitor **BP**, **labs**, and **weight**,

To help the heart self-regulate.

Lisinopril / Hydrochlorothiazide (Zestoretic)

ACE Inhibitor + Thiazide Diuretic Combination

A powerful pair in just one pill,
To help that **blood pressure** stay still.
Lisinopril blocks the **RAAS cascade**,
While **HCTZ** makes fluid fade.

The **ACE inhibitor** widens the lane,
By blocking **angiotensin's** tightening reign.
The **thiazide diuretic** works below,
Pulling **salt and water** with its flow.

Used in **hypertension**, strong and clear,
When a **single drug** won't bring it near.
Together they act in perfect sync,
One tells vessels to widen, one makes you pee in the sink.

But watch for that **dry and nagging cough**,
From lisinopril—it's common enough.
And **angioedema**—a serious sign,

Swelling the face, lips, tongue, or spine.

Dizziness may happen when pressure drops,
Or if **electrolytes** start doing hops.
Hyperkalemia from ACE's part,
But **hypokalemia** from thiazide's start.

Monitor **K**, **Na**, and **renal labs**,
Along with **BP** in detailed tabs.
BUN and **creatinine** rise with strain,
Especially when kidneys bear the pain.

Take it once a day, with or without meals,
But rise up slow—**orthostatic feels**.
Avoid **salt substitutes**, **NSAIDs**, and **lithium**,
All can clash and cause a problem.

Pregnancy warning: It's not advised—
May harm the fetus if it's prescribed.
So test before and always assess,
Switch if needed for safety's success.

Photosensitivity is a side note here,
So wear that sunscreen when skies are clear.
And watch for **gout** if they've had it before—
Thiazides can make uric acid soar.

Teach patients signs that raise red flags—

Swelling, **rash**, or **muscle crags**.

Ensure they know it's lifelong care,

To keep that pressure smooth and fair.

Loratadine (Claritin)

Second-Generation Antihistamine (H1 Blocker)

A **non-drowsy antihistamine**, smooth and clean,
It blocks **H1 receptors** without the scene
Of older drugs that cause a doze—
This one lets alertness stay composed.
Used for **allergic rhinitis** each spring,
When pollen and dust make noses sting.
Also relieves **hives** and itchy skin,
Urticaria—it works from within.

It **blocks histamine** released in flair,
So sneezing, itching, swelling—rare.
But it **doesn't cross the blood-brain line**,
So **sedation** is rare—most feel fine.
Take it **once a day**, with or without food,
The **24-hour** action keeps it smooth.
Teach patients not to take too much—
Overdose could bring a drowsy touch.

Side effects? Just a few:
Maybe **headache**, **dry mouth**, or feeling blue.

Sometimes **fatigue** or slight distress,

But mostly mild—patients report less.

Avoid combining with **alcohol**

Or other **CNS depressants** overall.

Though less sedating than first-gen peers,

It's good to check what else appears.

Watch **liver function** in those impaired,

And use with caution—be prepared.

For **elderly patients**, monitor close,

As they may be more prone than most.

It's safe in **pregnancy**, Category B,

But always check with the OB.

For kids, it's often used with ease—

Just adjust the dose to match their needs.

No need to taper—stop it clean,

When allergy season leaves the scene.

But for **chronic hives** that won't recede,

Daily use might still be the need.

Lorazepam (Ativan)

Benzodiazepine – Anxiolytic / Sedative-Hypnotic / Anticonvulsant

A **benzodiazepine**, fast and chill,
It calms the nerves and bends the will.
Used for **anxiety**, **seizures**, and **sleep**,
And **pre-op sedation** when patients weep.

It enhances **GABA**, the brain's "brake,"
Slowing things down for calmness' sake.
The **CNS depressant** class it joins—
It quiets the mind and relaxes the loins.

Anxiety disorders, **status epilepticus**,
Insomnia, or when panic gets treacherous.
It's strong, it's fast, but **short in stay**,
For **PRN** use—it's not for play.

Watch for **sedation**, **drowsy eyes**,
Respiratory depression is no surprise.
Especially with **opioids** on board,
That combo's one to not ignore.

Can cause **amnesia**, **low BP**,
Dizziness, or feeling unsteady.
And if used long, then suddenly stopped,
Withdrawal symptoms can make hearts drop.

Give **PO**, **IM**, or **IV** with care,
But **monitor vitals** when giving it there.
IV push? Go **slow and smooth**,
To help the CNS gently soothe.

It's a **controlled substance**, Schedule IV,
So track each dose, and don't give more.
Tolerance and dependence can occur—
Use short-term only, to be sure.

Don't mix with **alcohol** or CNS meds,
They enhance sedation and heavy heads.
And in **pregnancy**, avoid this train—
It crosses the **placenta** and affects the brain.

Monitor for **LOC**, **RR**, and **gait**,
And signs that the dose may not be great.
Teach patients **not to drive** or run,
Until they know how the med is done.

If **toxicity** comes into view,
Flumazenil can rescue you.

But slowly now—reversal can bring

Seizures back in a brutal swing.

Losartan (Cozaar)

Angiotensin II Receptor Blocker (ARB) – Antihypertensive

An **ARB**, not an ACE, but close in feel,
It blocks **angiotensin's binding deal**.
Instead of stopping its creation,
It blocks the **receptors**—a smart foundation.
Used for **hypertension** big and small,
And **heart failure**, to prevent the fall.
Also for **diabetic nephropathy**,
To help protect the kidney tree.

It relaxes vessels, drops BP down,
Letting blood flow all around.
Without that **ACE cough**—a bonus perk,
A quiet breath while it does its work.
But side effects still make their case—
Dizziness, **fatigue**, and slower pace.
Hyperkalemia may show its head,
So check those **K+ labs**, like I said.

Angioedema is still a risk,
Though lower than ACE, it still exists.

Hypotension can occur as well,
Especially in those not feeling swell.
Monitor **BP**, **renal labs**, and **weight**,
Check **BUN**, **Cr**, and **electrolyte state**.
Watch **potassium**, keep it tight,
Too much can cause a heartless fright.

No pregnancy—Category D,
This drug can hurt the fetus, see?
Stop it quick if pregnant, too,
And switch to something safer through.
Take **once daily**, with or without meals,
Same time each day improves the feels.
Avoid **NSAIDs** that raise the strain,
On kidneys already under the pain.

Tell patients not to use **salt subs**,
They're full of **potassium**, sneaky little clubs.
Teach signs of swelling, cough, or pain,
And how to rise slow—avoid the strain.

Losartan / Hydrochlorothiazide (Hyzaar)

ARB + Thiazide Diuretic Combination Antihypertensive

Two meds in one—what a clever plan,
To lower that pressure as best it can.
Losartan, an **ARB**, keeps vessels wide,
While **HCTZ** sends **fluid outside**.
Used for **hypertension uncontrolled**,
When one drug just won't take hold.
Together they help the system unwind,
By easing flow and clearing the grind.

Losartan blocks the **Ang II site**,
So vessels relax and pressure gets light.
HCTZ works in the **distal tubule**,
Losing **Na+ and water**, a classic rule.
Watch for **dizziness**, **fatigue**, and **thirst**,
Orthostatic hypotension may come first.
Photosensitivity can bring a burn—
So teach your patient, "Wear sunscreen, learn!"

Potassium levels can get wild—

Too high from ARB or **too low** and mild

From the **thiazide side** of the team—

So labs are key to keep things clean.

Monitor **BUN**, **creatinine**, and **K+**,

As well as **Na+** and **uric acid** each day.

Blood glucose can also rise—

So check in diabetics to avoid surprise.

No go in **pregnancy**—this drug's not safe,

Can **harm the fetus**, so don't chafe.

Teach your patient what to avoid:

Salt substitutes and **NSAIDs deployed**.

Take it **daily**, same time each,

With or without food—it's in your reach.

Encourage fluids (unless told not),

To help with balance and lessen clot.

Tell them to report **muscle pain**,

Swelling, **rash**, or anything strange.

Remind them not to **rise too fast**,

Or dizziness could knock them back.

Meloxicam (Mobic)

NSAID – Nonsteroidal Anti-Inflammatory Drug (COX-2 Preferential)

A **COX-2 selective NSAID**, smooth and slick,
It eases pain and works real quick.
For **arthritis**, stiff and sore,
It helps reduce **inflammation** at the core.
Used for **osteo** or **RA pain**,
It blocks the **prostaglandin chain**.
By inhibiting **COX**, it tones things down,
So joints can move without a frown.

Though gentler on the gut than some,
GI risk still doesn't succumb.
Can cause **bleeding**, **ulcers**, or **burn**,
So take with food—that's a good turn.
Headache, edema, or **dizzy spells,**
Ringing in ears or **BP swells**.
Can harm the **kidneys**, **heart**, and more,
So **labs and vitals**—always explore.

Monitor **BUN** and **creatinine** strong,

And ask if **NSAID use** has been long.

Check **CBC** and **liver tests**,

To keep an eye on organ stress.

Don't combine with other NSAIDs, please,

Or **anticoagulants**—that increases bleeds.

And don't mix with **ACE inhibitors** blind,

It may **reduce renal perfusion** in kind.

Avoid in **pregnancy**, especially late—

Closes ductus arteriosus at a dangerous rate.

So counsel women planning soon,

To switch off meds by the second trimester's moon.

Take it **once daily**, steady and neat,

Same time each day makes outcomes sweet.

Teach signs of **GI pain or blackened stool**,

Chest pain, SOB—no time to play cool.

Watch for **edema** or **BP up high**,

And **allergic reactions**—especially the eye.

Though rare, **SJS** or **TEN** can show—

Rash or blisters? Time to go.

Metformin (Glucophage)

Biguanide – Oral Antidiabetic Agent

A **biguanide**, first-line and wise,
For **Type 2 diabetes**, it takes the prize.
It doesn't boost insulin to rise—
It **lowers glucose** in other guise.
It **decreases hepatic glucose output**,
Slows absorption as it goes about.
It **improves insulin sensitivity**,
So cells take in glucose more efficiently.

It won't cause **hypoglycemia** alone,
Unlike sulfonylureas known.
But **GI upset** is quite the norm—
Diarrhea, nausea, cramps can form.
A rare but feared, though seldom seen,
Is **lactic acidosis**—harsh and mean.
Watch for **muscle pain, fatigue**, and **breath**,
Labored breathing could mean death.

Avoid in those with **renal decline**,
Check **GFR** to draw the line.

Under 30? That's a no-go zone,

30–45? Use caution alone.

Hold before contrast dye is used,

Or kidney function may be bruised.

Wait **48 hours**, then recheck labs,

Before restarting—no rehab flabs.

Take it with **food** to ease the gut,

Helps avoid the bathroom rut.

Give **once or twice daily**, as prescribed,

XR version keeps side effects mild.

It may cause **weight loss**—a bonus tip,

But add **exercise** for a healthy zip.

No alcohol binges while it's on board—

That raises **acidosis risk** ignored.

Check **A1C** and **glucose trends**,

And teach what each side effect portends.

Report any signs of serious strain—

Like **weakness, chills,** or **unexplained pain.**

Methylphenidate (Ritalin, Concerta)

CNS Stimulant – ADHD / Narcolepsy Medication

A **CNS stimulant**, quick and bright,
It brings **focus and attention** back to light.
For **ADHD**, it leads the pack,
Helping **impulse control** get back on track.

It blocks the reuptake—dopamine's ride,
And **norepinephrine** stays inside.
So neurons fire with better flow,
To help the brain stay in the know.

Also used for **narcolepsy**,
To stay awake and focused, see.
Short- and long-acting forms exist,
From **Ritalin** tabs to **Concerta**'s twist.

Expect some **appetite to fall**,
So **monitor weight**, especially in the small.
May cause **insomnia**, so dose with care—

Morning only—let them sleep fair.

Other effects? **Nervous mood**,
Headache, **BP up**, or altered food.
Tachycardia and **anxiety** too,
So vital signs must follow through.

Watch for signs of **abuse or misuse**,
This drug's a **Schedule II** with rules.
No automatic refills allowed—
So count and track it in the cloud.

May cause **tics** or **mood swings** in some,
And rare reports of **psychosis** come.
Assess for **suicidal thought**,
Especially when new scripts are sought.

Before you start, get **baseline weight**,
Height, **BP**, and **mental state**.
Then monitor each **follow-up**,
To keep the dosage level up.

Do not crush extended-release,
Give **whole and timed**—no quick release.
Capsules like **Metadate CD**
Can be sprinkled on food if that's more easy.

No caffeine, **alcohol**, or extra hype—

Stimulants clash with that type.

And if they stop it? **Taper slow**,

To avoid withdrawal's undertow.

Metoprolol (Lopressor, Toprol XL)

Beta-1 Selective Blocker – Antihypertensive / Antianginal

A **beta-blocker**, cardio-tied,
It keeps the **heart rate** low and wide.
Blocks beta-1, not beta-2,
So lungs are mostly spared from view.
Used for **hypertension, angina pain,**
Post-MI and **heart failure's** gain.
Also helps with **rate control** too—
In **AFib** and other rhythms askew.

It slows the **heart**, reduces strain,
So BP drops and hearts refrain.
But that can cause **bradycardia,**
Fatigue, dizzy, or **cold extremia.**
Hold the dose if pulse is slow—
Under **60**, let the prescriber know.
Watch for **hypotension**, lightheaded spells,
And **heart block** in those not well.

It may **mask hypoglycemia signs,**
Like shakiness or sweating lines.

So diabetics must be taught

That blood sugar checks should not be forgot.

There's **immediate** and **extended release**,

Toprol XL gives steady peace.

Take with food, especially Lopressor,

To increase absorption and make it more sure.

Taper slow—**do not quit fast**,

Stopping abruptly could be your last.

It can trigger **angina** or **MI**,

So always taper, don't defy.

Monitor BP, **pulse**, and more,

Especially when the patient's sore.

Check **ECG**, **weight**, and lungs,

And **signs of worsening HF** tongues.

Avoid with **calcium channel mates**,

Like **verapamil**—those compound fates.

Watch for **bronchospasm** in COPD,

Though it's beta-1, some crossover can be.

Montelukast (Singulair)

Leukotriene Receptor Antagonist – Antiasthmatic / Antiallergy

A **leukotriene blocker**, smooth and neat,
It helps the lungs and allergies meet.
Used for **asthma**, mild and tight,
And **seasonal allergies** day or night.
It blocks **leukotrienes** that inflame,
Preventing wheeze, not playing the game.
It **won't treat acute asthma flair**,
But **used daily**, it helps repair.

It helps with **exercise-induced wheeze**,
Taken **two hours before with ease**.
Also helps with **chronic rhinitis**,
Making airways less like tight fists.
Once daily dosing, in PM light,
With or without food—it's always right.
Chewables for kids are fruity and fun,
But don't take more than **one and done**.

It's generally safe, with **few side kicks**,

But some report **mood or behavior ticks**.

Agitation, **hallucination**, or **nightmares** bad—

Especially in children—so monitor, Dad.

Can also cause **headache** or **GI pain**,

Fatigue, fever, or **earache strain**.

Rarely **Churg-Strauss syndrome** too—

Vasculitis risk when steroids are through.

Not for rescue—don't be confused,

No use when acute symptoms are diffused.

That's when **albuterol** takes the lead—

This drug's for long-term asthma need.

Teach parents and patients what to see,

If mood or sleep shifts suddenly.

And always **assess respiratory trends**,

Like wheeze, cough, peak flow—it never ends.

Naproxen (Aleve, Naprosyn)

NSAID – Nonsteroidal Anti-Inflammatory Drug

A classic **NSAID**, strong and true,
For **pain**, **inflammation**, and **fever** too.
Blocks COX enzymes, both one and two,
So **prostaglandins** can't push through.
Used for **arthritis**, **sprains**, or **aches**,
And **dysmenorrhea**—menstrual shakes.
Also relieves **fever** and **gout**,
But **GI risks** you must point out.

Can cause **ulcers**, **bleeding**, **GI pain**,
So give with **food** to help restrain.
May lead to **heartburn**, **nausea**, **cramps**,
And **dark stools** or **coffee-ground vamps**.
Increased risk of **MI** or **stroke**,
Especially in patients who already broke.
So use the **lowest dose for the shortest time**,
To help the body and keep things fine.

Watch for **renal strain** as well,
BUN, **creatinine**—labs to tell.

Use caution with **ACE inhibitors** near,
It can stress the kidneys year to year.
May cause **fluid retention**, too—
Edema, **BP rise** out of the blue.
So monitor **vitals** and **daily weight**,
Especially in heart patients—it's not great.

Avoid in **pregnancy, trimester three**,
It may close the **ductus arteriosus**, you see.
And don't forget to **limit alcohol**,
It raises GI bleed risks overall.
Teach them signs they shouldn't ignore:
Chest pain, **weakness**, or **blackened floor**.
Tarry stool, or **bleeding gum**,
Means it's time to call—not stay numb.

Taken **twice daily**, with meals is best,
It keeps the gut calm and pain suppressed.
But **do not crush extended-release**,
Swallow it whole to keep the peace.

Olmesartan (Benicar)

Angiotensin II Receptor Blocker (ARB) – Antihypertensive

An **ARB** with strength and steady beat,
Olmesartan helps blood pressure retreat.
It blocks **Angiotensin II** from the site,
So vessels relax and **BP drops right**.

Used for **hypertension** control,
Protects the heart and kidney role.
Sometimes used when **ACEs cause cough**,
This ARB steps in to smooth things off.

It's taken **once daily**, with or without food,
Helps patients get into pressure-lowering mood.
But teach them to rise slow from their chair,
Orthostatic drops can catch unaware.

Side effects? A few, not wild:
Dizziness, fatigue, or **headache mild**.
But monitor for **hyperkalemia**,
And signs of **renal ischemia**.

Check **potassium, creatinine**, and **BUN**,
And keep a close eye as the doses run.
Avoid with **NSAIDs** or **lithium**, too—
They may cause levels to skew.

Though rare, it may cause **sprue-like enteropathy**,
With **chronic diarrhea** and weight loss pathology.
So if GI symptoms don't resolve,
A med switch might just be involved.

Not safe in pregnancy—that's a must,
It may harm the fetus, so in this we trust.
Switch to a safer class right away,
If baby plans are on the way.

Avoid salt substitutes—too much K,
Especially since this drug may sway
The body's natural balance through,
And **potassium overload** can ensue.

Omeprazole (Prilosec)

Proton Pump Inhibitor (PPI) – Antiulcer / Acid Reducer

A **PPI**, strong and sleek,
It shuts down acid—week by week.
It blocks the **proton pumps** in line,
To lower **gastric acid** over time.

Used for **GERD**, **ulcers**, and **esophagitis**,
And **Zollinger-Ellison**, though that one's the rarest.
It helps the gut to rest and mend,
And gives that burning pain an end.

Taken **once a day**—before meals is best,
So the stomach's primed for its acid rest.
Swallow whole—**don't crush or split**,
That coating's key to where it hits.

Side effects? **Headache, nausea, gas,**
Constipation, or **diarrhea** may pass.
Long-term use brings added concern—
Bone loss, fractures, or **B12's slow turn.**

Also risk for **C. diff colitis**,
Especially with age or antibiotic bias.
Teach patients signs they shouldn't ignore:
Watery stool, abdominal sore.

Check for **magnesium** running low—
Hypomagnesemia can start to show.
So monitor labs if used long-term,
And **supplement** if needed to confirm.

May **interact** with drugs that need acid,
Like **ketoconazole**, which gets too placid.
Also decreases **Plavix's might**,
So consult prescribers when both unite.

Taper if stopping, don't quit cold—
Rebound acid might take hold.
Lifestyle tips can help along—
No smoking, spicy foods, or coffee strong.

Ondansetron (Zofran)

Serotonin 5-HT3 Receptor Antagonist – Antiemetic

A **serotonin blocker**, smooth and sly,
It stops the **urge to vomit** high.
Blocks **5-HT3** right on cue,
In the **CNS and GI tract** too.

Used for **nausea**, both near and far—
From **chemo, radiation,** or **post-op scar.**
Also used in **pregnancy**, though off-label still,
To ease that morning sickness chill.

Given **IV, IM,** or **oral tab,**
Even **dissolving strips**—they're fab.
Give **30 minutes before** chemo starts,
Or **pre-op** dose to calm queasy hearts.

Common side effects? Not too many,
But **headache** and **constipation** show up plenty.
Also **fatigue,** or **fever slight,**
And a rare **rash** if things aren't right.

But here's the caution: **QT can prolong**,

So watch the **EKG** all along.

Especially if on **other meds**,

That stretch the beat and risk heart dreads.

Check **electrolytes**, like **K** and **Mg**,

Correct imbalances before you tag.

Those low levels plus Zofran's drift,

Can give a dangerous rhythm shift.

Teach patients not to chew or crush

The **ODT** form—it melts in a rush.

Place on tongue, let it dissolve,

No water needed—that's the solve.

Safe in **children**, **adults**, and **the old**,

But watch liver patients—go slow, be bold.

Max dose may be **lowered** there,

To prevent **hepatotoxic** scare.

Oxycodone (Roxicodone, OxyContin, Percocet)

Opioid Analgesic – Schedule II Controlled Substance

A **strong opioid**, full of might,
For **moderate to severe pain**, day or night.
It binds to **mu receptors** in the brain,
To block the signals that cause pain.
Used **post-op**, for **injuries**, or **chronic strain**,
But carry it carefully—**addiction** is a chain.
Short-acting or **extended-release**,
Both can help—but misuse won't cease.

Common side effects on the chart:
Constipation, right from the start.
Also **drowsiness, nausea,** and **dry mouth**,
And **respiratory depression**—watch going south.
It can cause **euphoria**, peace, or calm,
But it can also bring **misuse's** harm.
So monitor **mental status**, too—
And watch for signs of "taking more than due."

Hold if respirations drop too low—
Less than **12**? Then **don't let it go**.
Narcan (**naloxone**) must be close by,
In case of overdose—don't let them die.
Give **with food** to help the gut,
But warn them: **no alcohol**—keep it shut.
It **increases sedation**, so they must know,
To skip the drinks and take it slow.

Taper down—don't stop too fast,
Withdrawal symptoms can hit and last.
Sweating, **aches**, and **craving's** rise,
Teach them well—no big surprise.
It's **Schedule II**, locked and sealed,
So double-check and have it revealed.
Wasting doses? Document well—
Accountability is where we dwell.

Check **bowel function** daily too,
A **stool softener** may help them through.
And teach them how to safely store—
Out of reach, behind a locked door.

Pantoprazole (Protonix)

Proton Pump Inhibitor (PPI) – Antiulcer / Acid Reducer

A **PPI**, strong and wise,
It stops the **acid** that likes to rise.
By blocking the **proton pump** inside,
It calms the burn you'd otherwise hide.

Used for **GERD**, **ulcers**, and more,
Erosive esophagitis it helps restore.
Also helps in **Zollinger-Ellison**,
Where acid runs like a loaded gun.

Given **IV** or **oral** form,
It works best when taken warm—
That means **before meals**, once a day,
To help the stomach stay at bay.

Side effects? There's just a few:
Headache, nausea, diarrhea, too.
Long-term use may not be bright—
Low magnesium, fracture plight.

Risk of **C. diff** and **B12 low**,

If used too long, those signs may show.

So monitor labs if it's prolonged,

And watch for **muscle cramps** that don't belong.

Don't crush or split the delayed-release,

Let it dissolve in its coating piece.

Swallow whole for max effect—

That's how it protects and keeps things correct.

Taper it down if stopping the med,

To avoid **rebound acid** flaring instead.

Teach lifestyle tips to help the fix:

Like **eating slow, no spicy mix**.

Safe for **short-term hospital care**,

And often used with **NSAIDs** there.

To protect the gut from ulcer fate—

Especially in patients who medicate late.

Paroxetine (Paxil)

Selective Serotonin Reuptake Inhibitor (SSRI) – Antidepressant / Anxiolytic

An **SSRI**, calm and slow,

Paroxetine helps the **serotonin** flow.

Used for **depression**, **panic**, and fear,

Anxiety, **OCD**, and **PTSD** clear.

Also used for **PMDD**,

And **social anxiety**, shy and stressed.

Sometimes for **hot flashes**, too—

It has a wide range of things it can do.

It **blocks serotonin's reuptake train**,

So mood and calm can rise again.

But it takes a few **weeks to work**,

So teach them patience—not to shirk.

Common side effects in tow:

Nausea, fatigue, and sexual woe.

Weight gain, dry mouth, sweating, yawn,

And **drowsiness** lasting all day long.

Black Box Warning—don't skip this:

Suicidal thoughts can rise or exist.

Especially young folks, watch with care,

Check-ins and follow-ups must be there.

Serotonin syndrome is rare but real,

With **agitation**, **tremor**, or **feverish feel**.

Clonus, sweating, confusion, too—

If these show up, it's time to review.

Taper slow—don't stop too fast,

Or **withdrawal symptoms** might come in a blast:

Dizzy, irritable, zaps in the head,

Insomnia, tears, and dragging dread.

Avoid with **MAOIs**, wait **14 days**,

Or risk a crisis in bad ways.

Also use caution in **pregnant folks**—

Paroxetine's risks aren't just jokes.

Give **once daily, AM or night**,

Depending on if it brings **calm** or **flight**.

Can be taken with or without food,

Whatever keeps the stomach in a good mood.

Potassium Chloride (Klor-Con, K-Dur, Micro-K)

Electrolyte Supplement

A vital **electrolyte** the heart holds dear,
Potassium chloride—we give it with care.
It helps with **nerve**, **muscle**, and **heart rhythm**,
But out-of-range levels? Major symptom.
Used to treat or prevent **hypokalemia**,
When losses come from **diuretics** or **emesis anemia**.
It keeps **cardiac rhythms** strong and tight,
Preventing **PVCs** or arrhythmic fright.

But giving it wrong? That's a big no—
Too fast IV and the heart might go.
Never push IV—that's a code,
Always **dilute and drip** in the correct mode.
Oral forms include **liquid**, **powder**, or **tabs**,
Some are extended, so don't crush the slabs.
Take **with food** to help the gut,
It's harsh on stomach lining if kept in a rut.

Monitor for **GI upset, nausea, bloat**,
And check if pills can safely float.
Check labs before and during the plan,
You'll watch **K+**, and **renal function** if you can.
Normal **potassium** ranges tight—
3.5 to 5.0 is just right.
Too low, and cramps or weakness show,
Too high, and rhythms start to go.

Watch for signs of **hyperkalemia** creep:
Bradycardia, muscle twitch, or too much sleep.
Tall T waves on the ECG,
Means potassium's higher than it should be.
Don't give with **potassium-sparing meds**
Unless the doc is tracking the threads.
Avoid with **salt substitutes** as well—
They're loaded with K+ and could end in a spell.

Teach patients how to **take it right**,
Stay upright after dosing—don't lie tight.
With **plenty of water**, help it go down,
To protect the esophagus from a burn or frown.

Pravastatin (Pravachol)

HMG-CoA Reductase Inhibitor (Statin)

A **statin** med, heart-healthy and wise,
It helps bring **cholesterol** down to size.
It **blocks HMG-CoA reductase**,
The enzyme that makes cholesterol blaze.

Used to treat **high LDL**,
And raise that **HDL** as well.
Prevents **MI**, **stroke**, and more,
In patients with **cardiovascular score**.

Take it **once at night**, when the liver's awake,
Making cholesterol it needs to break.
Some forms can be taken **with food**,
But **Pravastatin** is flexible—choose the mood.

Watch for **muscle pain or cramp**,
Rhabdomyolysis sets up camp.
So teach your patients what to feel—
Weakness, dark urine, a muscle deal.

Can also harm the **liver's might**,
So monitor **AST**, **ALT** just right.
And don't mix with **grapefruit juice**—
Though not as risky here, best to reduce.

It's safer than some **statins in kind**,
Lower interactions, which is kind.
But still be cautious—**polypharmacy's** real,
Especially if **multiple risk factors** appeal.

Avoid in **pregnancy**—that's a must,
It can harm the fetus, break the trust.
Also not for **breastfeeding** folks—
Switch to safer meds or natural strokes.

Teach them it's **lifelong care**,
Cholesterol sneaks in unaware.
Lifestyle helps—**diet**, **exercise**,
While pravastatin keeps the lipids wise.

Prednisone (Deltasone)

Corticosteroid – Anti-Inflammatory / Immunosuppressant

A **corticosteroid**, strong and bold,
It **fights inflammation**, breaks the mold.
For **asthma**, **COPD**, **RA** flare,
Allergic reactions—it's everywhere.
Also used for **lupus**, **IBD**,
And **autoimmune** activity.
It **suppresses the immune system's spark**,
To help the body reset the mark.

Take it **with food**—that's rule one,
It's tough on **stomachs**, even when done.
Can cause **ulcers**, **bleeds**, or ache,
So GI protection's a move to make.
Short-term side effects come in quick:
Mood swings, insomnia, and feeling sick.
Increased appetite, fluid retained,
And **blood sugar spikes** not easily tamed.

Long-term risks are not so kind—
Cushing's syndrome may unwind:

Moon face, **buffalo hump**, and more,

Fragile skin, and bones that sore.

Watch for **infection** signs held back,

Because this drug **hides the usual track**.

No fever, yet infection grows—

So assess for subtle warning shows.

Monitor **weight**, **glucose**, and **pressure**, too,

And **electrolytes**, like **K** and **Na** that skew.

It can cause **hypokalemia** and **Na+ rise**,

And raise **WBCs**, but in disguise.

Taper slowly—never stop quick,

Or **adrenal crisis** could make them sick.

Teach to carry a **steroid card**,

And wear a bracelet—safety's not hard.

Not safe for **long-term in pregnancy**,

But short-term use may sometimes be.

Risk vs. benefit must be weighed,

And fetal health closely surveyed.

Pregabalin (Lyrica)

Anticonvulsant / Neuropathic Pain Agent – Schedule V

A **nerve pain med**, gentle and slow,
Pregabalin helps the signals flow.
Used for **seizures**, **fibromyalgia**, too,
And **diabetic neuropathy** coming through.
Also treats **spinal cord pain**,
And **post-herpetic neuralgia's** sting and strain.
Though it sounds like **GABA** in name and face,
It **doesn't bind GABA**—just holds its place.

It works by **calming calcium gates**,
In nerve cells firing fast like mates.
This slows the flow of pain's distress,
And brings the nervous system rest.
Dizziness, **drowsiness** top the chart,
So teach them safety from the start.
Avoid driving till they know,
How **sedation** and balance go.

Also may cause **weight gain**,
Blurred vision, **swelling**, or **mental strain**.

Dry mouth, **tremors**, or feeling blue,
Even **euphoria** in a rare few.
Risk for **dependence** is quite low,
But **Schedule V** means it still can show.
Use **caution in substance abuse past**,
And monitor how long it lasts.

Take it **twice a day** or **three**,
With or without food—it's flexible, see.
But don't stop it suddenly—no way,
Withdrawals can hit and ruin your day.
Watch for **angioedema**, rare but real—
Facial swelling that you must feel.
Teach patients to report at once,
Or airway swelling could pack a punch.

No alcohol, or go real light,
It **enhances sedation**—not a good night.
And monitor for **mood changes**, too,
Especially in those feeling low or new.

Propranolol (Inderal)

Nonselective Beta Blocker – Antihypertensive / Antianginal / Antidysrhythmic

A **nonselective beta blocker**, wide,
It calms the **heart** and eases the ride.
Blocks both **beta-1** and **beta-2**,
So it hits the lungs and heart tissue too.
Used for **hypertension** and **angina pain**,
And to **prevent migraines** in the brain.
Also treats **essential tremors** and fear—
Like **stage fright** when performance is near.

It slows the **heart rate**, drops **BP** down,
Calms **arrhythmias** when they come 'round.
But beta-2 means a lung effect,
So **asthma patients**—better redirect.
Can cause **bradycardia**, cold hands and feet,
Fatigue, **dizzy**, or faint in the heat.
Depression, **insomnia**, may show too—
So monitor mood as part of your view.

Hold if HR is under 60,

And always check **BP** for safety.

Watch for signs of **CHF**:

Weight gain, **crackles**, or **dyspnea left**.

It may **mask hypoglycemia** signs,

In **diabetics**, that can cross lines.

No **shakiness**, **sweat**, or racing pulse—

So blood sugar checks are a must.

Take it **with food** to slow absorption,

And reduce **GI upset** proportion.

Taper slowly—**never quit fast**,

Rebound HTN or **angina** could last.

Monitor ECG, **weight**, and **labs**,

And check for **edema** that sneaks or grabs.

Avoid **alcohol**, it boosts the block,

And may enhance the hypotensive shock.

Teach patients how to check their pulse,

And rise up slowly—don't convulse.

It's helpful but needs steady care,

With daily checks and symptoms to share.

Quetiapine (Seroquel)

Atypical Antipsychotic – Mood Stabilizer / Antipsychotic

An **atypical antipsychotic**, smooth and deep,
Quetiapine helps when thoughts won't sleep.
For **schizophrenia**, it leads the line,
And **bipolar swings** it helps align.

Also used for **major depression**,
As an add-on in tough progression.
It balances **dopamine** and **serotonin** too,
To calm the mind and shift the view.

It can cause **sedation**, strong and fast,
So take it **at night**, to help that last.
Also causes **weight gain**, quite a bit,
And **increased appetite** that's hard to quit.

Watch for **orthostatic drops**,
So rise up slow in gentle hops.
Dizziness, dry mouth, constipation,
All part of quetiapine's foundation.

Can raise **cholesterol**, **glucose**, and more,
So monitor **metabolic labs** at the core:
A1C, **lipids**, and **weight**, you see—
Especially with long-term therapy.

Black Box Warning—don't dismiss:
Suicidal thoughts in youth exist.
Also risk for **neuroleptic malignant syndrome**,
With **fever**, **rigidity**, and **mental gloom**.

Rare but serious is **QT prolongation**,
So **check the ECG** for confirmation.
And **leukopenia** may occur—
Monitor **CBC** to be sure.

Watch for **extrapyramidal signs**,
Like **tremors**, **restlessness**, awkward lines.
Though less than typical antipsychotics show,
It's still a risk you need to know.

Teach to never **stop abruptly**,
Withdrawal can come subtly.
Taper slow and plan ahead,
To keep the brain chemistry steady instead.

Avoid **alcohol** and **grapefruit juice**,
Both increase the drug's effect and use.
And caution with **other CNS depressants**,

To prevent a sleepy, risky presence.

Rivaroxaban (Xarelto)

Factor Xa Inhibitor – Anticoagulant

An **oral anticoagulant**, sleek and new,
Rivaroxaban prevents clots from breaking through.
It blocks **Factor Xa** in the clotting chain,
So **fibrin** can't form—and clots refrain.
Used for **DVT** and **PE** prevention,
Or **A-fib** stroke risk—worth a mention.
Also after **hip or knee repair**,
To keep those post-op clots rare.

It's taken **once a day**, often **with food**,
To boost absorption and set the mood.
No need for **routine INR**,
Unlike **warfarin**, it goes far.
But bleeding risk is always there,
So teach them what to watch and share:
Bruising, **bleeding gums**, or **blood in stool**,
Or sudden weakness—don't play cool.

There's **no reversal** that's widely known,
Though **andexanet alfa** may be shown

In certain cases when bleeding's severe—

Still, prevention is key right here.

Avoid with **NSAIDs** or **aspirin crew**,

They raise the risk of bleeding too.

And **liver or renal** impairment states

Require adjusted dosing rates.

Don't skip doses, take on time,

Clot risk climbs with missed pill crime.

And don't stop suddenly without plan—

Stroke risk returns faster than you can scan.

Teach patients to report all meds,

Even **herbals** or **supplement threads**.

Like **St. John's Wort** can interfere—

It lowers drug levels year to year.

Watch for signs of **bleeding inside**,

Like **black tarry stools** or **eyes gone wide**.

Hematuria, **dizzy**, or **low BP**,

All could mean internal bleed, you see

Rosuvastatin (Crestor)

HMG-CoA Reductase Inhibitor – Antilipemic Agent (Statin)

A **statin drug**, bold and clean,
Rosuvastatin keeps vessels serene.
It blocks **HMG-CoA's reign**,
To lower **cholesterol** in the vein.
Used to drop that **LDL**,
Raise **HDL**, and **triglycerides** quell.
Prevents **stroke**, **MI**, and plaque buildup,
Keeps the arteries smooth and up.

Take it **once a day**, food or not,
Evening preferred, but timing is a flexible spot.
Swallow whole, don't crush or split—
That coating's there to make it fit.
Side effects? A few might show:
Headache, **GI upset**, or energy low.
But the big ones that you must know—
Rhabdomyolysis creeping slow.

Watch for **muscle pain**, weakness, or cramp,
Dark urine, **fatigue**, or a heavy stamp.

Check **CK levels** if symptoms appear,
And hold the dose if side effects steer.
Also keep an eye on the **liver**,
AST and **ALT** can start to quiver.
Especially early, when therapy starts,
Monitor labs and liver parts.

Risk for **proteinuria** is rare but real,
So **kidney labs** help track the deal.
And **glucose may rise**, so monitor too,
Especially if **diabetes** is already in view.
Avoid in **pregnancy**—it's Category X,
Stops cholesterol the fetus expects.
So contraception must be tight,
While on this drug, both day and night.

No grapefruit warnings here apply,
Unlike some statins that amplify.
But still check other **meds they take**,
To avoid interactions and a mistake.

Semaglutide (Ozempic, Wegovy, Rybelsus)

GLP-1 Receptor Agonist – Antidiabetic / Anti-Obesity Agent

A **GLP-1 agonist**, smart and sleek,
Semaglutide helps balance peak.
It mimics hormones from the gut,
To **lower glucose** and **shut hunger shut**.

Used in **Type 2 diabetes** care,
And for **weight loss** in those who dare.
Ozempic helps with sugar control,
While **Wegovy** helps weight loss goals unfold.

It **slows gastric emptying**, curbs appetite,
Helps insulin release stay just right.
Reduces **glucagon**, trims the spike,
Keeps post-meal sugar from jumping the bike.

Taken **weekly** via **subQ shot**,
In **abdomen**, **thigh**, or **arm**—pick your spot.
Start **low and go slow** to avoid the wave,

Of **nausea, vomiting,** and **gut misbehave.**

Oral form? Yes, **Rybelsus** is new—
Take **on an empty stomach** with water true.
Wait **30 minutes before you eat,**
And don't take with meds or juice or meat.

Side effects that may appear:
Nausea, diarrhea, or **belly unclear.**
Fatigue, dizziness, or **mild reflux,**
But usually fade as the body adjusts.

Watch for **pancreatitis pain**—
Severe upper belly, sharp and plain.
Gallbladder issues may arise,
With **pain under ribs** or **yellowed eyes.**

Black Box Warning: cancer seen
In rodents' **thyroid medullary gene.**
So **avoid in patients** with thyroid ties,
Like **MEN2** or **cancer** that still applies.

Monitor **glucose, A1C,** and **weight,**
And signs of **hypoglycemia's fate,**
Especially if combined with more—
Like **sulfonylureas** that lower the score.

Not for **Type 1** or **DKA,**

This isn't insulin—it works another way.

Teach lifestyle change for best success,

Diet, **movement**, and **stress-less**.

Sertraline (Zoloft)

Selective Serotonin Reuptake Inhibitor (SSRI) – Antidepressant / Anxiolytic

A trusted **SSRI**, steady and clean,
Sertraline helps the mood stay serene.
It boosts the **serotonin** in your brain,
To ease **depression**, **anxiety**, and pain.
Used for **MDD**, **OCD**, and **PTSD**,
Panic disorder, and **social anxiety**.
Also helps with **PMDD** strife,
Balancing hormones and emotional life.

Taken **once a day**, **morning or night**,
With or without food—it's patient's right.
But start **low and go slow**, as is wise,
To minimize side effects that may rise
Watch for **nausea**, **drowsy days**,
Dry mouth, **diarrhea**, or foggy haze.
Sexual dysfunction—a common gripe,
Insomnia or dreams that feel too ripe.

Black Box Warning—know this well:

SERTRALINE (ZOLOFT)

Suicidal thoughts in youth can swell.
Monitor mood and **energy shift**,
Especially early or after a lift.
Rare but serious is **serotonin storm**—
Fever, **agitation**, **clonus** form.
If paired with **MAOIs** or meds not clean,
This syndrome's risk becomes more seen.

Never stop it **suddenly**,
Or **withdrawal** might come heavily:
Zaps, **dizzy**, **mood swing**, **tears**,
Flu-like symptoms, anxious fears.
Takes **weeks to work**, not just one,
So teach that healing's rarely done
Without commitment to the ride—
And support close by their side.

Safe for long-term in most folks,
But caution with **liver** or **seizure** pokes.
Use in **pregnancy**? Sometimes yes,
But weigh the risks—discuss and assess.

Simvastatin (Zocor)

HMG-CoA Reductase Inhibitor – Antilipemic Agent (Statin)

A **statin med** that fights the fight,
Simvastatin lowers **lipids** right.
Blocks **HMG-CoA** in the liver's core,
So your body makes **cholesterol** no more.
Used for **high LDL**, and more—
It helps prevent **stroke**, **MI**, and **plaque galore**.
It also raises **HDL** a bit,
And drops those **triglycerides** that won't quit.

Take it **once daily**, in the **evening hour**,
That's when your liver's in statin power.
With or without food is fine,
But teach them **bedtime's** the statin sign
Watch for **muscle pain** and **cramp**,
Rhabdomyolysis can set up camp.
Teach them to report **darkened pee**,
Or **weakness** that's new and shouldn't be.

Check **liver labs**—**AST**, **ALT**,
Especially early in therapy.

Watch for signs of **liver stress**,
Like **fatigue, yellow skin**, or GI mess.
Not safe in **pregnancy**—Category X,
So always assess before you Rx.
Breastfeeding? Also not advised,
This drug must be safely minimized.

Avoid **grapefruit juice**—it's bold,
It **raises statin levels** more than told.
That increases risks you don't need,
Like **toxicity** that can mislead.
Watch for **drug interactions** high—
Like **amiodarone** or **gemfibrozil** nearby.
They can raise the statin's power,
And cause muscle aches to flower.

Lifestyle still matters—don't forget,
Diet, exercise, goals well set.
This med is strong, but not alone,
Healthy habits must be grown.

Sitagliptin (Januvia)

DPP-4 Inhibitor – Oral Antidiabetic Agent

A **DPP-4 inhibitor**, smooth and sly,
Sitagliptin helps **blood sugar** not run high.
It works by **boosting incretin flow**,
So **insulin rises** when glucose grows.
It **lowers glucagon** when you eat,
So **post-meal sugars** can't compete.
Used for **Type 2 diabetes care**,
To gently nudge the levels there.

It's taken **orally once a day**,
With or without food—either way.
But don't use it in **Type 1** scenes,
Or for **DKA**—it won't intervene.
Most tolerate it really well,
But some **side effects** still may swell:
Headache, runny nose, or **sore throat**,
Upper respiratory infections get a note.

But watch for **pancreatitis pain**—
Severe, sharp, and won't abstain.

Left upper quadrant or radiates back,
If that appears, it's time to act.
Can rarely cause **joint pain** that's strong,
Or **allergic reactions** that last too long.
Stevens-Johnson (though rare) may show—
With **rash, blisters,** or **skin that glows.**

Check **renal function**—that's a must,
Because kidneys clear this drug's dust.
Lower the dose when GFR's down,
To avoid buildup that could drown.
It's often used in **combo form**,
With **metformin** or others in norm.
But if combined with **insulin or secretagogues**,
Watch for **hypoglycemia** logs.

Teach patients signs of sugar lows,
Shaky, sweaty, or **slurred prose.**
And always pair it with lifestyle grace—
Diet and **exercise** in place.

Spironolactone (Aldactone)

Potassium-Sparing Diuretic / Aldosterone Antagonist

A **potassium-sparing diuretic**, kind,
Spironolactone calms the aldosterone grind.
It blocks that hormone's salty grip,
So **Na+ is lost**, but **K+ won't slip**.
Used for **heart failure**, **cirrhosis**, too,
And **hypertension** that won't subdue.
Also treats **hyperaldosteronism**,
And **acne** or **PCOS**—hormone prism.

It helps the body **drop excess fluid**,
But keeps **potassium**—that's why it's suited
For folks who can't afford to lose
More **K+** through peeing than they choose.
Side effects may include a few:
Hyperkalemia—watch the view.
Check for **muscle cramps**, **tingling**, or **slow HR**,
Tall T-waves on ECG raise the bar.

Also causes **gynecomastia** in men,
And **menstrual changes** now and then.

Breast tenderness, impotence, fatigue,

Are hormonal shifts you may need to league.

Take with **food** to ease the gut,

Helps avoid that nausea rut.

Best in **AM** to avoid late pee,

Though it's milder than loop diuretic pee.

Avoid **salt substitutes**—they're full of K,

Which can push the heart the wrong way.

And don't mix it with **ACE inhibitors**,

Or **ARBs**—you'll raise the risk for triggers.

Monitor labs: K, BUN, Cr,

To see how well the kidneys are.

And weigh the patient every day—

Sudden gains mean fluid stays.

Pregnancy? It's **Category C**,

Not first-choice med in maternity.

So assess if someone's trying soon,

And weigh the risks before they swoon.

Sumatriptan (Imitrex)

Serotonin (5-HT$_1$) Receptor Agonist – Antimigraine Agent

A **triptan drug**, fast and tight,
Sumatriptan brings **migraine** relief to light.
It **stimulates serotonin 5-HT$_1$**,
To shrink those vessels once the pain's begun.
Used for **acute migraine** attacks,
And **cluster headaches** that come in packs.
But it **doesn't prevent**—don't take it each day,
It's for **when the aura** won't go away.

Comes **oral**, **nasal**, or **subQ pen**,
Fast delivery to feel better again.
Inject in **thigh** or **arm** subcutaneously,
Relief may come within an hour, easily.
Side effects include **chest pressure**,
Or **tightness** patients often measure.
May feel like **heaviness, neck or jaw pain**,
That mimics a heart issue—but it's not the same.

Still, rule out **cardiac risk** before,
Since **vasoconstriction** is at its core.

Avoid in those with **CAD**,

Stroke, or **uncontrolled HTN**, you see.

Can cause **tingling**, **flushing**, or **dizzy**,

And **fatigue** that makes them feel less busy.

May also cause **nausea** or feel odd—

But usually fades once it's trod.

Serotonin syndrome is a concern

If with **SSRIs**, **SNRIs** in turn.

Look for **fever**, **agitation**, or **clonus** move—

And act fast if symptoms prove.

Can take **1 dose**, and if pain remains,

Repeat in **2 hours** if still migraine.

But don't exceed the **daily cap**,

Or rebound headaches might just snap.

Teach them not to drive too fast,

Until they know how long effects last.

And avoid with **ergot meds** in view—

Must wait **24 hours** between the two.

Tamsulosin (Flomax)

Alpha-1 Adrenergic Blocker – BPH Treatment Agent

A **selective alpha-blocker**, smooth and slow,
Tamsulosin helps that **urine flow**.
Used in **BPH**—the prostate swell,
It helps the bladder empty well.

It **relaxes smooth muscle tone**
In **prostate** and **bladder neck** alone.
So patients feel less strain and stress,
Less **urgency**, and **retention** mess.

Not for **blood pressure**, though it may
Cause **orthostatic drops** along the way.
So teach them how to **rise up slow**,
To keep the **dizzy spells** on low.

Take it **once a day**, **30 minutes post-meal**,
Preferably **same time** to seal the deal.
Do not crush or chew the shell,
It's **extended-release**—that won't end well.

Side effects include **nasal stuff**,
Headache, **back pain**, and **feeling rough**.
Ejaculation issues may show too,
It's **retrograde**—so don't misconstrue.

May cause **floppy iris** during eye ops,
So tell the **surgeon** before the drops.
Even if you stopped it weeks ago,
This **intra-op risk** is good to know.

Monitor BP, though not the goal,
Because the alpha-blocking takes a toll.
No need for labs, but always assess
For **urinary relief** or **retention stress**.

Not used in **females**, as a rule,
Though off-label may stretch that tool.
Usually safe, well-tolerated,
But **first-dose hypotension** is often stated.

Tizanidine (Zanaflex)

Centrally Acting Alpha-2 Adrenergic Agonist – Muscle Relaxant

A **muscle relaxant**, calm and clean,
Tizanidine helps relieve the scene.
For **spasticity**, it's often given—
MS, **spinal injuries**, movement driven.
It acts on the **central nervous zone**,
Where **alpha-2 receptors** are known.
It **inhibits motor neuron fire**,
So tense, tight muscles can retire.

Given **oral**, short-acting dose,
Works **fast**, but doesn't always last most.
Take it **up to three times a day**,
But spacing doses the right way.
Side effects are common here:
Drowsiness, **dry mouth**, or brain not clear.
Hypotension and **dizzy drop**,
So monitor **BP**—and don't just stop.

Liver enzymes may elevate,

So monitor **AST/ALT** straight.

And **renal clearance** plays a role,

Dose adjust if kidneys aren't whole.

Avoid **alcohol**, CNS depressants too—

Sedation increases and function skews.

Also caution with **CYP1A2 drugs**,

Like **ciprofloxacin**, which raises shrugs.

Can cause **hallucinations** in rare case,

Or a weird **psych state** to take place.

Taper down if stopping the med,

Or **rebound hypertension** may be ahead.

Not for long-term if not required—

Use when **short bursts** are desired.

And teach them not to drive too fast,

Until they know how long effects last.

Topiramate (Topamax)

Anticonvulsant / Antimigraine Agent

A brain-calming med with multiple roles,
Topiramate helps meet seizure goals.
Also used to prevent **migraine pain**,
And sometimes for **binge eating**, **weight loss** gain.
It modulates **GABA** and **glutamate**,
To keep the firing neurons straight.
It blocks **Na+ channels** in the brain,
And tames electrical signals' strain.

Used for **epilepsy** and **Lennox-Gastaut**,
And for **mood disorders**, it's sometimes sought.
Helps with **alcohol** and **drug withdrawal**,
And **off-label** uses? There are a haul!
Side effects? Let's talk clear:
Drowsy, dizzy, or cognitive smear.
They may say "I feel slow or spaced,"
Or like their **words have been displaced**.

Watch for **kidney stones**—hydrate well,
And **metallic taste** some patients tell.

Weight loss can be a helpful trait,

But **anorexia** risk may elevate.

May cause **tingling in hands or feet**,

Called **paresthesia**—not so sweet.

And can raise **ammonia**, rarely seen,

Leading to **encephalopathy** mean.

Can cause **metabolic acidosis**,

So check **bicarb** if symptoms focus.

Monitor **eye pressure** too, just in case—

Angle-closure glaucoma can show its face.

Take **with or without food**, but note—

Swallow whole, don't crush or coat.

Taper if stopping, never just cease—

Seizures may spike, not decrease.

Pregnancy? There's a warning to heed—

It may cause **cleft palate** to proceed.

So in those planning to conceive,

Discuss all risks before they believe.

Tramadol (Ultram)

Opioid Analgesic – Schedule IV

A **pain reliever**, gentle and light,
Tramadol treats **moderate pain** just right.
Not as strong as full opioids seem,
But still **binds mu-receptors** in the scheme.
It also blocks **serotonin and norepinephrine** reuptake,
Which helps with pain—and mood's own ache.
That dual action makes it unique,
But side effects still make us speak.

Used for pain that's **chronic or new**,
But not for **severe** or **breakthrough** too.
Comes in **IR**, **ER**, or **combo pills**,
But **watch the dosing**—to prevent chills.
Can cause **drowsiness, dizzy, nausea, dry mouth**,
And **constipation**—like opioids south.
Seizure risk goes up with dose,
Especially with SSRIs close.

Serotonin syndrome is a rare scare,
If mixed with **MAOIs**—beware!

Watch for **fever**, **tremors**, or **agitation**,
That calls for immediate medication cessation.
Though weaker, **dependence** can still form,
And **misuse potential** is far from norm.
So it's **Schedule IV**, not over-the-counter,
Track each dose—don't let it flounder.

Avoid in **renal** or **hepatic decline**,
Dose must be changed to stay in line.
Also not for kids post-tonsil,
Risk of **respiratory depression** is no thrill.
Take it **with or without food** okay,
But teach to **avoid alcohol** every day.
And if they're driving or using machines,
Be sure they know what that really means.

Taper slowly if taken long,
Stopping fast could go all wrong.
Withdrawal may look like flu gone wild—
Chills, nausea, or mood unstyled.

Trazodone (Desyrel, Oleptro)

Serotonin Antagonist and Reuptake Inhibitor (SARI) – Antidepressant / Sedative

A **SARI** med—dual in tone,
Trazodone works in a sleepier zone.
It **blocks serotonin reuptake** just a bit,
And **antagonizes 5-HT$_2$**—that's its split.
Used for **depression**, though not first-line,
But it's loved for **sleep**—that effect is fine.
It calms the mind, slows thoughts that race,
And helps with **insomnia's restless case**.

Take at bedtime, once per night,
Its **sedation** can dim the light.
May also help with **anxiety**,
Though its role there's used off-label, you see.
Common side effects on the chart:
Drowsiness, dizzy, and **dry mouth** start.
Orthostatic hypotension too—
So **rise up slow** is key to do.

Can cause **headache**, **blurred vision**, weird dreams,

And **GI upset** in mild extremes.
Weight changes, or **sweating** mild,
Are effects that might be reconciled.
A rare but serious event:
Priapism—yes, it's what it meant.
A painful **prolonged erection** state—
Teach patients to seek help—**don't wait**.

Use **caution in elderly**, risk is steep,
Fall risk rises if they're half-asleep.
Can cause **arrhythmias**, QT prolong,
So monitor **EKG** before too long.
Don't mix with **MAOIs** at all,
And **serotonin syndrome** can call—
Especially when paired with meds
That **boost serotonin** in similar threads.

Taper slowly if they've been on it long,
To avoid **withdrawal** that hits strong.
It's not controlled, but still go slow—
Respect the med and symptoms that show.

Triamcinolone (Kenalog, Nasacort, Aristocort)

Corticosteroid – Anti-Inflammatory / Immunosuppressant

A **corticosteroid**, local and strong,
Triamcinolone helps where things go wrong.
It fights off **inflammation, swelling**, and **itch**,
Whether **topical, nasal,** or **joint**—it's rich.
Used for **eczema, rash,** and **psoriasis pain**,
Or **inhaled** for **asthma**, to calm the strain.
It also comes in a **nasal spray**,
To treat **allergies** the inflamed way.

In **injections**, it soothes **arthritis flare**,
Or **bursitis**, or **keloids** that won't repair.
It **suppresses the immune system**, too,
So symptoms stop when steroids are due.
But steroids have side effects, too—
So here are some to share with you:
Thinning skin if used too long,
Bruising, stretch marks, feeling wrong.

With **nasal** or **inhaled**, you might see:

Hoarseness, sore throat, or **oral thrush debris**.

So teach them to **rinse** when puff is done—

Prevents that yeast from having fun.

With **injections**, watch for mood swings loud,

Or **fluid retention** in the crowd.

Hyperglycemia may come in tow,

So **monitor glucose** if levels grow.

Don't use on broken skin or eyes,

And not for **long-term use**, if wise.

Occlusive dressings may enhance the soak—

So check for thinning skin that's broke.

Pregnancy? Topicals are often fine,

But assess the dose and frequency line.

For **systemic use**, weigh the risk,

Short-term is safest if they must persist.

Teach to **taper slowly** if taken by shot—

The **adrenal glands** forget a lot.

But with creams or sprays, just ease them out,

When the flare is gone—no need to shout.

Venlafaxine (Effexor, Effexor XR)

An **SNRI**, bold and true,
Venlafaxine lifts the **mood** and view.
It boosts both **serotonin** and **norepinephrine**,
To help the **fog of depression** thin.
Used for **MDD**, **anxiety**, **panic**, and more,
Social anxiety and **hot flash** lore.
It treats the mind and nervous state,
But must be taken **regularly—not late**.

Comes in **immediate** or **extended release**,
The **XR form** gives symptoms peace.
Take with food, and at **same time daily**,
To keep the blood levels steady, not wavy.
Side effects that often show:
Nausea, **dry mouth**, and **sweating glow**.
Insomnia, **drowsy**, or **loss of drive**,
And sometimes **increased BP** may arrive.

So check their **pressure** now and then,
Especially in **higher XR mg** pen.

Also **headache, dizzy, blurred-out sight**,

And **sexual dysfunction**—a common plight.

Black Box Warning—please don't miss:

Suicidal thoughts in young adults exist.

Monitor closely in the early phase,

Especially during those first few days.

Taper **slowly**—this one's key,

Withdrawal symptoms come rapidly:

Brain zaps, nausea, crying fits,

Tremors, vertigo, anxious bits.

Serotonin syndrome—rare but real,

If used with other meds that deal.

Watch for **fever, tremor, agitation**,

And seek fast help without hesitation.

Caution in **hepatic** or **renal stress**,

Lower doses may be best.

And avoid with **MAOIs** near,

Give **14 days** to stay clear.

Warfarin (Coumadin)

Vitamin K Antagonist – Oral Anticoagulant

An **anticoagulant**, classic and strong,
Warfarin's been around so long.
It blocks **vitamin K-dependent clotting**,
Which keeps the **coagulation** from over-spotting.

It inhibits factors **II, VII, IX, and X**,
Also proteins **C and S**—complex friends.
Used to prevent or treat **clots** with pride:
DVT, PE, or **A-fib** wide.

Stroke prevention is the goal,
In those whose clots may take a toll.
But warfarin's strength comes with a twist—
You need to **monitor labs** on the list.

Watch the **INR**, keep it tight,
2 to 3 is the usual sight.
Too low? A clot could still appear.
Too high? Then **bleeding** is near.

Takes **several days** to fully start,

So use **heparin bridge** if you're smart.

And if you need to **reverse the dose**,

Vitamin K helps the clotting host.

Teach patients to stay **diet aware**,

Leafy greens have **vitamin K** to spare.

Don't stop eating them—keep it **steady**,

Big swings in intake aren't ready.

Frequent INR checks are a must,

To make sure levels stay in trust.

Same time daily, with or without food,

Routine makes things go smooth and good.

Side effects? **Bleeding**, first of all—

Gums, **urine**, **stool**, or sudden fall.

Bruising easy, bleeding long—

Report those signs when something's wrong.

No NSAIDs or **aspirin** on the sly,

Unless the prescriber gives the why.

And tell the doc all meds they take—

Even herbs or teas they make.

Pregnancy? Nope! It's a no-go,

Fetal defects have been shown to grow.

Use safer options if baby's in view,

Warfarin risks are more than a few.

OTHER TITLES IN THE MADE EASY SERIES

Geriatrics Made Easy
Emergency Care Made Easy
Critical Care Made Easy
Human Growth & Development
Maternal & Newborn Made Easy
Mental Health Made Easy
Organic Chemistry Made Easy
General Chemistry Made Easy
Pediatrics Made Easy
Med-Surg Made Easy, Vol 1
Med-Surg Made Easy, Vol 2
Microbiology Made Easy
Nursing Skills & Procedures
Pathophysiology Made Easy
Nursing Assessment Made Easy
Nutrition Made Easy
Anatomy & Physiology Vol 1
Anatomy & Physiology Vol 2

Pharmacology Series

Pharmacology Made Easy Vol 1
Pharmacology Made Easy Vol 2
Pharmacology Made Easy Vol 3
Oncology Meds Made Easy
Cardiac Meds Made Easy
Endocrine Meds Made Easy
Pain Meds Made Easy
GI Meds Made Easy
Respiratory Meds Made Easy
Critical Meds Made Easy
ER/ICU Meds Made Easy
Neuro Meds Made Easy
Psych Meds Made Easy
Pediatric Meds Made Easy
OB/GYN Meds Made Easy

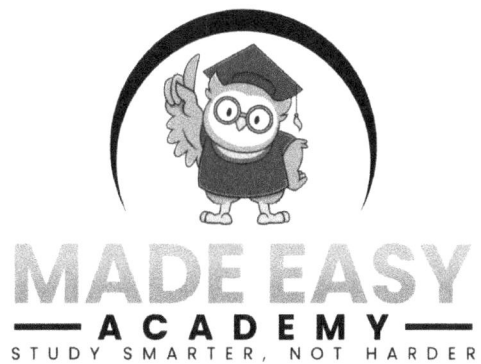

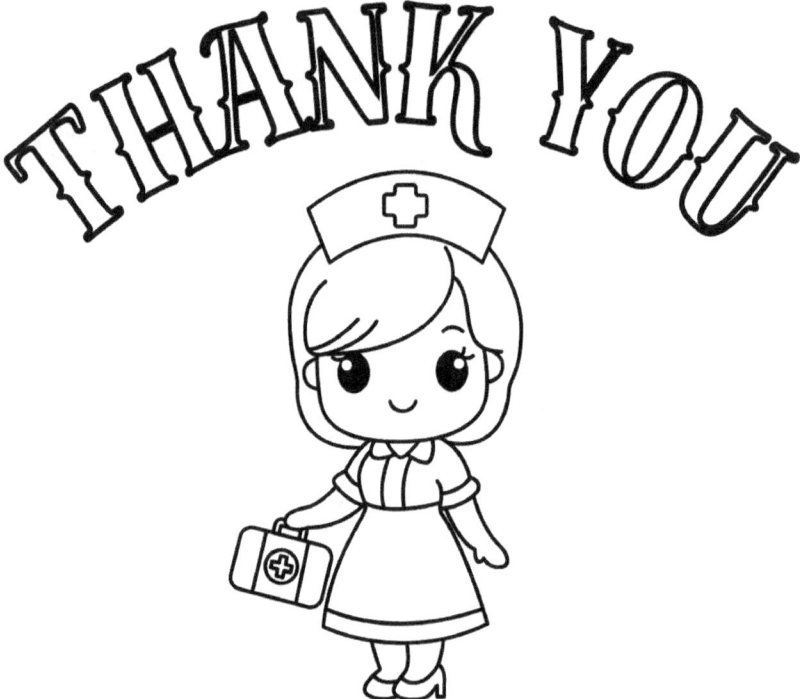

for getting this book and for making it all the way to the end!

Before you go, I wanted to ask you for one small favor. Could you please consider posting a review? Because posting a review is the best and easiest way to support the work of independent authors like me.

Your feedback will help me a ton!

Click **Here** or Scan the QR code below!

www.ingramcontent.com/pod-product-compliance
Lightning Source LLC
Chambersburg PA
CBHW071020240526
45469CB00006BD/2014